Runner's World

ADVANCED INDOOR EXERCISE BOOK

Runner's World
ADVANCED INDOOR EXERCISE BOOK

by Richard Benyo
and Rhonda Provost

Runner's World Books

Library of Congress Cataloging in Publication Data

Benyo, Richard.
  Runner's World advanced indoor exercise book.

  (Instructional book; 7)
  Bibliography: p.
    1. Physical fitness. 2. Exercise. I. Provost,
  Rhonda, 1948- . II. Title. III. Title: Advanced
  indoor exercise book. IV. Series.
  GV481.B482   613.7   81-17835
  ISBN 0-89037-167-9 (spiral)   AACR2

© 1982 by
Richard Benyo and
Rhonda Provost

No information in this book may be reprinted in any form
without permission from the publisher.
Runner's World Books
in conjunction with
Anderson World, Inc., Mountain View, Ca.

Contents

Dedication		vi
Introduction I		vii
Introduction II		ix
1.	Just How Fit Is Fit? (or, Survival of the Fittest)	1
2.	Going Nowhere Fast, Slow Or In-Between	53
3.	Keeping All Systems Flexible	87
4.	Spinning Your Wheels	119
5.	Floor Games	161
6.	The Muscle Beach Party Gang Meet Slim-Person	193
	About the Authors	231
	Recommended Reading	233

Dedication

For Dr. Dick Berggren, who in his own unique way made this book possible, which is to either his credit or his eternal damnation, depending on which side of the fence you lean. And for Super, often long-suffering, always philosophical.

Introduction I

Some prognosticators of the social condition are predicting that within a decade, two at the most, everything we want to do, we will be able to do in the home. They credit/blame this trend on the incredible advances in electronics, and they feel that many other industries will follow suit so that the average American will eventually spend a minimum of time outside.

Theoretically, cable TV will give us all the entertainment we used to go out to the movie theaters to enjoy, minus those hassles we won't have to worry about finding gum stuck up under our seats, pay ninety-five cents for an "economy size" box of Good & Plenty, or wait in line. It will be less expensive, we won't have to burn gas for the car to get us there, be distracted by the young couple behind us with the crying baby or be bothered by the adolescent couple in front of us discovering the birds and the bees and studying human anatomy on Saturday nights in the dark. Home computers and the recent tremendous advances in communications will enable many people who now commute to work to stay at home and do their jobs through television screens and monitors.

Such advances are putting us perilously close to missing out on what makes everyday life interesting: the chance of being mugged, or hit by a car or bus, or breathing sulfuric acid fumes from auto exhausts, or having a pigeon—or worse yet, a sea gull—use us for target practice. For everything gained, something must be given up.

We will likely also give up much of the "traveling for fun" that we do. Instead of driving three days, fighting traffic and sleeping in strange motel beds to get to the south rim of the Grand Canyon, we can get comfortable with a can of beer in the living room, draw the drapes from in front of the wall-sized screen, push a button, and feel as though we were on a hang glider, sailing out

INTRODUCTION

over the Canyon, and experiencing it like we never could have in person.

Sounds like science fiction, but such a lifestyle isn't that far away. It also sounds as though I'm being cynical about it, which I probably am, but I don't mean to be. There will be a big advantage in the saving of natural resources, but TV screens certainly take the adventure out of life, and might turn us into creatures too paranoid to step outside the door. (If all of us were kept in our rooms for a few years, though, that might allow nature to begin repairing some of the damage we've done to her.)

One of the very positive trends in this new emphasis on our homes as centers of activity is the growing line of products being developed for indoor exercising.

While there is a trend for Nautilus-type equipment in formal gymnasium and health spa use to become larger, bulkier and seemingly more complex, on the other side of the spectrum there is a trend toward development of lightweight, portable, easy-to-use equipment for the home.

Some of the equipment coming along is extremely functional and downright clever. In our original volume in this instructional series, *The Runner's World Indoor Exercise Book*, we discussed the fact that there are many people who feel inclined to begin exercising but who are too intimidated to go to a gym or to rush out the door to go running down the street as a full-blown jogger.

Many people who could benefit greatly from a regular exercise program are very tentative about embarking on one, for various reasons. They may feel self-conscious about their body, which they feel has degenerated from the generally accepted impression of the physically fit. Or they may feel uncertain about how to exercise properly, because they may have had a very inferior physical education program in high school or college, or perhaps no program at all. They have no idea how to get started.

There are as many reasons as there are people for feeling less-than-enthusiastic about rushing out to a health spa or out onto the streets to work up a sweat. Doing it in the comfort of their own home, where they can feel at ease and where it is no one else's business what exercises they do or how many of them, would make a world of difference.

Even for the person who frequently goes to the local health club to work out, there can be inconveniences. There are just some days when there's no time to jump in the car and rush over to the health club to do an exercise, so the workout for that day is skipped. Not good.

The solution for many people is to invest in one or more pieces of home exercising equipment. In this volume, I'll be looking at some of the available equipment, and subsequently setting up programs for some of those devices.

I must be frank about this: I, like a lot of outdoor exercisers, came to using the home equipment bearing a longstanding prejudice against it. I've had some fairly bad experiences on similar equipment over the years (which I'm sure you'll gather from some of the stories opening the various chapters), but went away from the experience this time with a real appreciation of how far and how fast some of the equipment has evolved.

Without further ado, let's get into some heavy breathing.

—Richard Benyo
Palo Alto, California
December 1981

Introduction II

Many risk factors affect us daily, resulting in disease and disability. Life is a gamble, waiting to see which disease or illness will lay us low. Some of these factors are beyond our control, such as pollution, genetics and highway hazards. However, we do have some control over the vagaries of life—our everyday behavior for one. Despite the fact that all of us are subjected to risk factors, not all of us become ill. That's partly luck. But most of us who do not become ill have personalities characterized by commitment, control, and a desire to challenge life's roadblocks.

A new, healthy view of the human physical condition is emerging, one more factor to put the odds on our side. The sensitivity, resiliency and recuperative powers of the human body are finally being acknowledged. My mailbox is continually stuffed with brochures advertising symposiums and workshops on such topics as stress management, assertiveness, hypnosis, wellness, cardiovascular health, nutrition, and so on. The hospital where I am employed conducts "support group" meetings on a regular basis. This has all resulted from medicine's recent recognition that these topics and others, including exercise-related matters, play a major

INTRODUCTION

role in determining who remains healthy. The medical establishment is finally shifting its emphasis from symptomatic to preventive medicine. Completely eliminating stress, which instigates many current medical problems, is an impossibility now, unless we return to the cave. However, teaching people a variety of ways to cope with stress is a viable alternative. And frequent exercise for all ages is highly recommended for reducing stress, increasing fitness, and personal performance. Dealing with stress in this way is just one example of preventive medicine at work.

Regular exercise enhances our potential for fitness and the three components to fitness are strength, endurance and flexibility. Most forms of exercise promote more of one of these components than the others. Bicycling, for example, emphasizes endurance, but not strength and flexibility.

In this book we attempt to provide you with the opportunities to enhance all three fitness components. One appealing aspect of these programs is that you are set on a course of self-improvement. More is gradually asked of you as you progress, but if you have done all the exercises you'll have no problem meeting the increasingly demanding challenges.

So we have established that exercise is good for you. Okay. But why *advanced exercises*? You shouldn't have undue anxiety over the word "advanced." By definition, the word "advance" means *to move forward*. Being advanced merely stresses being beyond elementary or introductory, and you are beyond elementary or you would not be reading this book. "Advanced" emphasizes being beyond others in progress and development. My only alteration to the above definition is that the emphasis rests in being beyond *yourself*, not others. After all, you are exercising for your own benefit, not someone else's.

So why *advanced exercises*? First, it can be fun, especially when you see and feel results that reinforce your motivation to continue. Second, the fact that you are embarking on an advanced exercise program reflects the fact that you have already achieved a certain level of fitness. You are perhaps positively addicted (no pun!) to exercise. Third, you may have accepted the challenge to see just how much you are capable of. You will need control of both your body and mind. This element of control spills over into other areas of your life. It can build character and commitment.

In our original volume, *The Runner's World Indoor Exercise Book*, we began with simple exercises and progressed to the more

Introduction

complex. Much significance was attached to matters such as warming up and cooling down. This volume assumes that you are at a certain level of achievement. You mastered the basics: Relax, Be Gentle, Be Patient. Although you have a new base from which to begin, realize that the basics still apply.

Since achievement and fitness maintenance come with regular exercise, and you have made the initial commitment, you want to get to work on an activity plan for healthful living that will endure for a lifetime. The equipment and exercises in this book provide you with more avenues to explore on that journey to fitness. Our assumption is that you are capable of expanding your abilities even farther. We hope that you will not stop here. After all, there is still swimming, cycling, racquetball, tennis, running . . .

—Rhonda Provost
Palo Alto, California
December 1981

1

Just How Fit Is Fit? (or, Survival of the Fittest)
by Richard Benyo

Why are so many Americans fat and out of shape?

A frequently posed question, that—even in an age when our country is caught up in a fitness revolution. At least we are constantly told there is a fitness revolution.

The popular press would have us believe that the fitness revolution is here and it is going to cure all of our ills and give us longer and more fulfilled lives and make us feel younger—and isn't it wonderful....? The popular press uses terms like "tip of the iceberg" when describing all the people running and bicycling and going to health spas and walking and skipping rope and rollerskating. A term like "tip of the iceberg" fits nicely into a news story about fitness because it hints that the reporter has many additional facts about the subject that he is not divulging, that there is a virtual underworld of fitness addicts surreptitiously making the country fit without its knowledge and against its best efforts to resist.

Bull's balls!

The "fitness revolution" is still merely a whimper. The people you see running and bicycling and walking and whatnot are in no way the "tip of the iceberg." They *are* the iceberg. There is no fitness underworld as there was an underworld in Al Capone's Chicago or in France during its occupation in World War II. Those you see huffing and puffing, sweating and straining along the highways and byways of America are all we've got.

The majority of Americans are still sublimely out of shape and most of them are overweight for their age, height and sex.

It would be nice to say that they are not at fault for their condition. And, perhaps by really stretching a point, we can do that. (Not that it is going to change the fact that they're out of shape and overweight, of course.) Or at least we can convince them that it is only 95 percent their fault.

The other 5 percent is society's fault, the fault of changing times, and the fault of bad habits and attitudes. Which still leaves us with the heavy and profound realization that it is still 95 percent our own fault if we're fat and out of shape. Some consolation, huh? What would W.C. Fields say about such a situation? "Ah, yes. There is an excuse for being ugly. You can blame your parents. But for being fat *and* ugly, oh no, that'll never do." We're not here, though, for W. C.'s comments or public consolation. We're here for action—and for information needed to direct that action.

But before we begin dealing with the 95 percent of the problem, which is each individual's attitude, let's examine a history of voluntary ill health.

Let's go back in time 100 years.

If we could put you in a time machine and do just that, when the door opened on another century in the good old US of A, what would you see? Besides the fact that everyone would be wearing clothes markedly different from your own, that paved roads would be unheard of, that there would be no telephones (or telephone lines) anywhere, and that there would be no cars, trucks, gas stations, fast-food places or malls to service the very mobile society we know, there would be something else very much in evidence by its absence: *fat*.

Oh, you might see one or two fat people out of each hundred, but you would soon realize something very revealing about that one or two. In almost every instance, you would be able to accurately guess his occupation—or at least accurately guess his status in the society.

Because, you see, the fat people would have to be people who were:

1. Involved in a profession that gave them little physical activity, such as a banker, lawyer or shopkeeper.

2. At least moderately wealthy; consequently there would be little need for hard, physical labor.

3. A non-professional, poor person currently unemployed but getting plenty of food from somewhere.

This is not to say that all bankers, lawyers, shopkeepers, wealthy people or unemployed (but still eating) poor people were fat. Many of them weren't. Some bankers had so much tension in their lives (and still do) from worrying about other peoples' money, its safety and how to make it grow, that they worried calories away. Some wealthy people were just skinny by nature because one or both of their parents had been skinny and had passed this svelte body-type along to them.

Most of the people in this country a century ago earned their living from, as the term goes, "the sweat of their brow." What that means, quite simply, is that they worked their asses off to put bread and meat on the table.

The husband worked the loading dock, the mines or the fields for 10, 12, even 15 hours a day. At home, the wife worked hard scrubbing floors, doing the wash and making the meals. (There were no easy-to-wipe linoleum floors, no Maytag washing machines that never needed repairs, and no microwave ovens.)

The majority of Americans worked long, hard, physically demanding hours for six and often seven days out of the week.

Their compensation was that they lived in America. Every American (save the Indians, and ultimately, even them—) was either an immigrant or a descendant of an immigrant who had fled his native country for one of several reasons. One major reason was because his former country had a lower standard of living. Another was famine.

America, whatever its faults when they arrived, *was* the land of plenty, at least in three areas: land, opportunity and food.

Just as the promise "My kids are going to get the chance for the education I never had" rang in America a generation or two ago, so the promise many a parent made a century or more ago was similar: "I'm gonna make sure my kids don't ever have to go to bed hungry the way I had to in the old country."

Through hard work, ingenuity, and a land that lent itself to the service of the supper table, America became the best-fed country in the world, a cornucopia.

And Americans, because of their hard, manual labor, had appetites that were ready to make short work of the promised plenty.

Except for the occasional hard times, the family's mother set a table that would choke a shark. It's no wonder everyone sat around Sunday afternoons after a good dinner belching at each other. I grew up in a mining community, among families of immigrants from Ireland, Germany and Czechoslovakia, and a Sunday meal invariably threatened to snap the legs of the table—meat, bread, potatoes, two or three other vegetables, milk, dessert.

For a hard-working person, the immensity of that Sunday meal was fine and dandy. The father, a coal miner, might burn up 5500 calories a day at hard labor. The mother, doing work around the house from sunup until well after sundown, might burn 4500 calories. For such active lives, large quantities of calories were needed (as fuel) to keep them going at their accustomed speed. As you can't drive a car that gets 20 miles per gallon 100 miles on four gallons of gas, so the hard-working father and mother of a century ago needed the large volumes of food to live and keep going.

But, unfortunately, they kept eating the same quantities, even as society introduced many labor-saving devices into the home, and most of the hard jobs were either phased out or were at least partially accomplished by machines. The American male's job-description changed radically. He was no longer swinging a heavy pick at a vein of coal 300 feet underground from before sunup until suppertime. The coal mines had modernized; now he was working in a factory where he pressed buttons to let machines do the heavy work. When he arrived home from work, because the "Big Feed" had been deeply ingrained, he was suddenly a man burning 2500 calories a day and still eating 5500, the same amount his father had consumed. Meanwhile, the housewife devoured 4500 calories a day, as her mother had, while burning a mere 2100.

Using the car analogy again, we now had a car capable of 10 miles to the gallon going 20 miles but on four gallons of gas. The extra gas had to go somewhere; that somewhere was right in the car's tank. The extra calories the American man and woman were putting away had to go somewhere, too.

On arrival in the body, calories stand around all in a group, like recruits in the army, expecting to be called upon to expend themselves for the good of the greater body. Unfortunately, many are eaten, but few were called in modern man. For the rest of the calories, it means taking up residence because there's nothing else for them to do at the moment. For every 3500 of those little buggers who take a vacation in a human body, one pound of useless fat is added.

The problem, then, is a rather simple one. Simple but heavy. You can drop pounds by not eating as much, or by doing something physical to use up the calories.

When you are heavy, of course, you are usually sluggish. And when you are sluggish, you have a more difficult time moving about. And when you have a difficult time moving about, you are going to tend to refrain from taking part in any kind of exercise or activity.

There's a dual problem here, of course. There is overweight *and* there is being out of shape. If you are in shape, you tend not to be overweight. But just because you lose weight (by dieting) doesn't mean you are automatically in shape.

Because much of what a dieter loses is not fat but muscle tissue, the ideal situation for a heavy person is to begin a safe and sane exercise program to burn off excess calories while toning and strengthening the body.

And by overweight, we're not referring to the grossly overweight, the blimp. A person can be overweight by ten pounds and feel sluggish.

Excess fat is merely relative. What bothers you may not bother someone else. Each person, by taking a good look at himself, can tell if there is some excess fat needing trimming and some muscles needing toning.

In many instances, a good exercise program can make dieting unnecessary. When I weighed 207 pounds, I was eating and drinking less than I am today when I'm in the 155-165 pound range; but then I wasn't engaged in anywhere near the physical activity that I am today.

And the great thing about the kinds of activities available is that they do not have to be advertised or even hinted at. Exercise programs done in the privacy, intimacy and comfort of your home can be just as effective as those done outside on city streets. And you are less likely to get run over by a car.

Once a goodly number of Americans embark on a regular program of indoor exercises, it will make the media a lot more believable when they throw around terms like "tip of the iceberg." At that point the runners and cyclists and hikers will be backed by an underworld engaged in undermining the fat and out-of-shape image that has been too long and too common on the American scene.

THE HEART OF THE MATTER

Death is something that is inescapable. It strikes down the rich and the poor, the weak and the strong, the careful and the reckless. The line goes that death and taxes are the only things you can be sure of in life. Some people, though, through legal maneuvering and loopholes, manage to avoid taxes. No one has managed to avoid death, unless we are ready to believe the stories of Dracula. But people seem to be constantly working on possible methods to do just that.

Death, the theory goes, is a disease. And, like other diseases, it can be cured. The theory has something to do with the gradual wearing down of cells. If the cells could be kept healthy, the great scientific minds believe, aging and death could be held back for extremely long amounts of time. Even if a cure is found for aging, death is still inevitable. If it becomes possible to extend the average person's life to 200 years, it is merely relatively longer than the three quarters of a century that many people are living today and the 480 years average age for inhabitants of the planet Jigygiyt. Life would still eventually lead to death—it would just be a more protracted trip.

Even if you were somehow to find a pill that could bestow immortality, there is no guarantee that you would be immortal. You could fall down a flight of stairs and die, or have a traffic accident, or become bored with immortality and commit suicide. There is a whole catalog of ways human beings can die, very few of them pleasant and none conducive to life.

The sincere hope of most people is that they will live a good and happy life, reach old age, and die in their sleep. Very few of us receive all our wishes so beautifully packaged. Death eventually catches up with each of us and takes its toll, which it begins extracting, a little at a time, from the moment we are born.

Very few of us are comfortable with the thought of death. In fact, there is a reluctance to even talk about it. We don't want to be reminded of our mortality. We even invent cute little phrases to help us avoid facing it. Uncle Mort didn't *die*, he *passed away*. Hell, people pass gas and pass a bar exam or pass out at the bar, but they don't "pass away." Uncle Mort, who used to chase the neighborhood kids away from his apple trees with a five-foot-long switch and who lived rather morosely with his two rat-chasing cats in a run-down shack at the end of town, went to bed one cold night and the debris in his chimney, which he was too lazy to clean out, caused carbon monoxide from his wood stove to fill the shack, and he *died* from it. He didn't *kick the bucket* or *check out* or *go on a trip from which he'll never return*. He just plain up and died. The next morning they found him stiff as a dead mackerel and after a few years the several apple trees near his shack, because of lack of care, went bad, so the neighborhood kids no longer needed mean old Uncle Mort to chase them away from the almost-ripe fruit. No one knows what happened to the cats; they just wandered off as cats will do. But three years after his death, when the city got around to plowing under his eye-sore of a shack, they found a Mason jar under the floorboards that contained nearly $100,000 and a little will of sorts that left it all to his cats. That's real dead, because they could never find the cats to award the money. Which was okay by the town, because they didn't need that kind of publicity.

People are currently becoming obsessed with death. Not in a morbid, Edgar Allan Poe sort of way, but on two fronts.

On the first front, they are trying to come to grips with the very concept of death. They are contemplating their own death and the death of people near them. I suppose a good way for them to get started in this contemplation of death is to begin using the word *die* instead of using phrases that are supposed to soften it. Death is a fact of life. We must all ultimately face it. And, in the game of checkers we play with death, we must be realistic enough to know beforehand that we'll always lose. The most we can do is get a few kings and keep our checkers moving in patterns that will at least temporarily confuse Death and put off the inevitable for a few more months...or rounds. That, perhaps, is one of man's more silly but still noble traits: he won't admit defeat even when it stares him down from across the cosmic checkerboard. In that small matter, three cheers for man, the most stubborn of animals!

The second way that man is becoming obsessed with death is by becoming obsessed with maintaining the highest level of life. This involves his current rush into exercise and health. There is more perspiration than ever being sprayed around the health spas, homes and highways and byways. More people are doing more grunting and groaning for their own good than in all of history, and that's terrific.

As we discussed in the previous section, the health craze is due to a growing awareness of our expanding midsections as a result of eating at a 1910 level in a present-day world that does not demand that amount of calories. It is an attempt to extend life. Or, at the least, it is an attempt to make what life there is a bit more enjoyable by being able to take a more active part in it.

This is a terrific movement that is doing more for the health of the country as a whole than all the posters and health-oriented official pushes combined. There is a very vital awareness that we do not have to be victims of our environment and lifestyle.

The battle has only been joined at this point, however. As we already discussed, the body of the iceberg is a huge one that needs a good, swift kick to get it moving to the surface of awareness—and action. The very positive aspect of this awareness is that, after so many years of confusion and inactivity relative to health and fitness, steps are being taken, even if tentatively.

The trip will, by no means, by an easy one. We are still uncertain about much of what is killing us before our time.

Heart disease, in its various forms, accounts for more than half of the adult deaths in the United States each year.

If we could significantly cut into the number of deaths from heart disease, we could take several giant steps toward ending deaths other than from old age. We could lead more active, fulfilling lives if we could rid ourselves of the disabling spectre of heart disease.

One of the problems is that we do not really understand heart disease. Discuss heart disease with the average person and his reactions are all very stereotypical. Mention "heart attack" and check his reaction. "Heart attack. Well, that's when someone's heart stops and they die," he might comment. "Unless, of course, he's near medical help and can be revived." It is seen almost like a drowning.

I must admit, my idea of what a heart attack was closely paralleled all the stereotypes and oversimplifications in the book. A few years ago, if someone had said to me, "Tell me what happens during a heart attack," my answer would have been something like this:

"Well, in a heart attack, the heart, which is a large muscle, just cramps up and sort of gives up. It becomes erratic, skips a beat or two, tries valiantly to keep going, but just gives up and the body stops living because it is no longer receiving nourishments and oxygen from the bloodstream."

In most heart attacks, this is an erroneous explanation. In fact, in almost all cases, this is dead wrong.

The hearts of most people who die of a heart attack are quite capable of carrying them through many more years of life. The problem is not with the heart. A large, powerful muscle, the heart is usually a victim of gradually closing arteries and veins. The arteries and veins become clotted with "plaque," a substance that builds up on their walls because of bad diet and little exercise. Plaque acts like grease sticking to a window. Leave it there for a while and it'll harden and stay. Add more grease, and it'll build up on top of the old, dried gook. Over a number of years, you've got a pretty stubborn mess that has built layer upon layer. Within the arteries, that same buildup contributes to their closure.

So, the heart is doing its work, but it is facing a great deal of resistance. It's like a spigot on the side of the house trying to push water through a garden hose that's got a crimp in it. What does get through does so with a tremendous amount of pressure because there is so much more water building up behind it also wanting to get through that small opening. Sound like high blood pressure? It is.

We don't want to slow down the examination of exercise by getting into a complicated explanation of how your heart works under normal conditions, and how it is restricted from working under abnormal conditions. It is valuable, when contemplating an advanced exercise program, however, to know exactly what the exercise is likely to do for you—and to you. What it will do is further strengthen your heart, it will begin breaking down the built-up plaque (by producing high-density lipoproteins, which surge through the arteries and literally begin scrubbing the built-up plaque in them, just as you might use a window-washing solution like Windex to break up the gook that's been building up on the window we mentioned).

Before going farther on this topic of exercise, and before getting farther into this chapter, on being tested to see where you are physically before upping your commitment to exercise, let's look at a startling revelation:

Heart disease in the United States is not so much a medical problem as it is a sociological problem.

But it's plaque building up on the walls of the arteries that causes a heart attack. *You just said that!*, you'll contend. Right. But the plaque has to be caused by other factors, and those factors come from a fount of woes that are very much grounded in sociologically induced habits.

Let's take a look at the most common factors contributing to heart disease, including indicators of heart problems:

    1. Systolic blood pressure

    2. Diastolic blood pressure

    3. Cigarette smoking

4. Cholesterol
5. Low-density lipoproteins/high-density lipoproteins
6. Cholesterol/high-density lipoproteins
7. Triglycerides
8. Blood glucose
9. Percentage of body fat
10. Stress-tension index
11. Amount of physical activity
12. Maximal oxygen consumption
13. S-T index (EKG abnormality)
14. Family history of heart disease
15. Age

The commonly accepted theory has been that most (if not all) of these factors were events caused by nature, by life in general, and over which we had no control.

The fitness revolution, however, has changed a lot of that thinking—at least among those experts who don't have their heads stuck in the sand.

The overwhelming majority of these factors do not happen as a matter of course, or through the intervention of nature. They are not as inevitable as the tides and the rising of the sun. Most of the factors are merely symptoms of sociology and heredity.

Heredity?

But, you'll contend, only number 14, "family history of heart disease," can be classified as heredity.

Not really. The factors that can often be traced to heredity are numbers 1, 2, 3, 4, 5, 6, 7, 8, 9, 10, 11, 12, 13 and 14.

If you stop and think about our discussion in the last section on how Americans have tended to get fat because they now eat too much, the pattern will emerge quite clearly.

Most of our habits in life are formed at youth, and are directly affected by our family (heredity) and our environment.

A family with a history of high blood pressure may perpetuate that history because the home life is filled with tension (screaming and shouting at each other over the supper table), exercising very little or not at all, therefore putting on weight and from that, having a high concentration of cholesterol. This leads to a preponderance of low-density lipoproteins, which contributes to plaque building up on the walls of the arteries. The resulting smaller passages force the blood pressure to increase to maintain sufficient flow—or high blood pressure.

It is the rebel offspring, the one who breaks away from the negative traditions, who escapes the majority of the factors contributing to heart disease. Very few offspring genuinely rebel to the extent that they break away from the heredity of their upbringing. They may move out of the house, but they take much of the learned heredity with them and pass it along to future generations.

When we began this section, we talked in terms of sociology. And sociology is very closely akin to heredity, especially of the learned heredity we are discussing. All we need to do is take the family learned heredity and broaden it to include the neighborhood or the entire community.

Let's consider some hypothetical examples in order to protect the guilty and avoid spending a lot of time in court arguing libel cases.

THE FALL AND RISE AND FALL OF THE CHANESKY FAMILY

The Chanesky family hailed from Central Europe. In the early part of this century, their country came apart due to political and economic upheaval. Al and Erma Chanesky with their three-year-old son, Gabe, fled the country. After a difficult and dangerous trip through Europe, they managed to get a boat from France to New York. They suffered through the indignities of Ellis Island, and headed inland, hoping to find some peace and stability.

Down to their last *rebniks*, they settled where they were because they could afford to go no farther. The town they settled in was Coal Haven, Pennsylvania. The principal business of the town was mining, and shipping that hard coal to coal-burning furnaces in Philadelphia and New York. The coal was shipped in two ways: on rails, and down canals on barges, which were broken up at their destination, their wood being sold as firewood and for building.

Al Chanesky took the first job that came to hand, which was working in the mines. He was used to hard work and was not adverse to the long hours in the mines. Erma set up house in one of the company-owned row homes. The community of 2754 souls had other families from the country the Chanesky family had fled. There were also immigrant families from Germany and Ireland.

Each group pretty much kept to itself; each group had its own church and its own social functions; each group was suspicious of the other because of the long-standing tensions between their countries in Europe, despite the fact that the men of the town worked elbow-to-elbow six days a week in the mines.

Al's day began at 3:30 when Erma woke him from a sound sleep. He had long since given up trying to scrub the ingrained coal dust and splinters from his rough hands where they looked like tatoos, but he splashed some water on his face and changed into his working clothes, which Erma had cleaned by hand the night before and hung up to dry. Erma made his breakfast, which was his largest single meal of the day—bacon, a half-dozen fried eggs and fried potatoes that had been reworked from leftover baked potatoes. He wiped his plate clean with thick, homemade bread, and drank several cups of black coffee. If there was any cake left from the previous day, he would eat a piece of that, too. By 4:30 he was heading for the mine shaft, his lunch pail swinging from his right hand, a cigarette hanging from his lips. The lunch pail was filled with sandwiches of roast beef and homemade bread, another piece of cake and a jar of warm soup. The cigarette would be his last until he came out of the mine at 4:00 in the afternoon. It was dangerous to smoke in the mines; an open flame could set off an explosion from trapped gas. Miners who had to have their tobacco were allowed to use chew tobacco in the mines, but there was no smoking.

While Al worked hard in the mine, Erma took care of the house, cleaning it by hand, hauling water from a spigot a block away. She made all the clothes for her family, washing them by hand and hanging them to dry on sagging clotheslines that ran like spider webs behind the line of row homes in which she lived. Her day was a thing of constant movement, between washing and cleaning, sewing and baking, cooking and cleaning up again. Time with Gabe was precious to her, but the child took care of himself, finding amusement around the house and in the dirt street in front of the house. He was a sociable child and played well with the neighborhood children. Erma's amusement for the day came from talking with her neighbors over the low fences between their yards in the back of their homes; they talked over the fences while they hung wash to dry. Their hands and faces were reddened and stung by the cold weather and by the hot weather; their bodies became hard. Although they did not become wealthy as they had originally half-hoped when they left their homes to come to America, neither did they starve. They put a little aside for calamities and for their old age, but they ate well, the food being brought in through the company store from the prosperous Pennsylvania Dutch farms not far away. There was a constant supply of smoked hams, plump poultry, Pennsylvania Dutch baked goods such as shoo-fly pies and pastries, scrapple, fruit (especially apples), cold meats, potatoes (which, like apples, could be easily stored in earthen cellars for use all year long), other vegetables in season, honey, grains, flour, sugar and dairy products. When Erma Chanesky needed food she could walk, with her son on one arm and her basket on the other, to the company store, pick up what she needed, and the store manager would mark it down in "the book," from there to be deducted from her husband's pay from the company.

For those willing to work hard, America was the land of plenty. When the day was done, Al's supper would be ready at 5:00, giving him time to wash some of the coal dust from his body and to blow some of it from his nose into his constantly soiled handkerchief. Erma kept a huge supply of handkerchiefs in his top bureau drawer in the bedroom. Al had already had a cigarette on his walk home, and after a hearty supper with his family, he would go out on the back porch to have another cigarette (you did not smoke in the home) and perhaps to contemplate the stars for a few minutes. After spending a few minutes with his son, he would take the short walk down to either the community's barroom (also owned by the mine company) or to his church-affiliated social club for a few beers with the boys, perhaps a game or two of darts, some talk and some good-natured plotting to organize a union to show those mine company bastards who they were dealing with, a few more cigarettes, more talk, and then he'd walk home, perhaps a bit more unsteadily than he'd left, but still very much his own man. Perhaps he'd engaged in a session or two of arm-wrestling, for strength was a great measure of a man in that environment, and Al Chanesky was no weakling. He would arrive home by the time young Gabe had been put to bed, and he would spend a bit of time with Erma relating the events of the day. Erma would tell him about what Gabe had done during the day, about what the neighbor women had had to say (this was the best form of gathering local news before each little town developed its own newspaper), and about what she had been doing. Al would relate a few incidents from his day and would perhaps tell Erma about something that had happened at the bar that evening. By 9:00 they would have gone to bed, Al stepping out onto the back porch for one last cigarette before retiring.

As Gabe grew, he would get some schooling (likely not beyond the eighth grade, and likely in a religious-affiliated school), because his parents felt it was an opportunity he should have even if it meant some sacrifices to pay for his education. Upon graduation, however, Gabe got a job shoveling ashes at the ash bins on the railroad, where the coal-burning locomotives emptied their furnaces. He lived at home for several years after going to work, but became more and more uncomfortable there because of his father's late-night coughing spells. He loved his parents, but his father's increasing bouts with colds and his occasional spitting up of black spittle into his handkerchief made him uneasy. Like his father, he enjoyed a cigarette and a glass of beer with the boys. He also enjoyed the hearty meals his mother put on the table for both of them. His work in the train yard did not consume the number of calories that his father's hard coal mining did, however, and he found himself becoming heavier than his father. He was putting on more weight, but the black lung that had begun consuming his father was causing ill-health and weight loss.

By the time his father died his slow, body-racking death, Gabe had begun his own family two blocks away. He had a wife, like his mother, and three children. Gabe and his wife took in his mother after her husband died because she had no place else to go. Social Security was just beginning, and had no provisions yet for Erma Chanesky, nor was there an acknowledgment of black lung as a disease that would have qualified her for a disability pension. Gabe, although he did not work for twelve hours a day in a cloud of coal dust that would be drawn into his lungs, had begun coughing for no apparent reason. He smoked more and drank more and in 1934 he was involved in a movement to organize a union, which cost him his job. He had to hussle, holding down two jobs and working twelve to fifteen hours a day to support his family. In 1942 he was sitting on the back porch after supper, very, very tired, talking with his oldest son. His son offered him a cigarette, but for one of the first times his son could remember, Gabe refused it. A pained expression came over Gabe Chanesky's face. He moved his 227 pounds uneasily in the rough chair. His son's face expressed concern. "Your mother's beans are giving me gas again," he said, a pained smile on his face. His son smiled back, turned to look at the sky for a moment, and turned back in shock when he heard his father's surprised gasp for breath. His father's mouth opened but nothing came out except a gurgling sound. Before he could leave his chair to help him, Gabe Chanesky had slumped forward, dead of a heart attack.

Fifteen years later, on the same back porch, in a newer chair, Gabe's own son would suffer a similar heart attack at the age of 38. He had been a clerk in the company that had at one time owned the town. He had been nearly as heavy as his father, but on a smaller frame, and his habits were similar to his father's: he had smoked, he had eaten his fill, his joy had been his family and his twice-weekly bowling sessions with the boys. His stress came from working to send a son through college and trying to argue away the guilt of his one daughter becoming pregnant at age 17 and running away to California—and he felt the town would never forgive him for it. His job offered the satisfaction of a paycheck and nothing else. He was literally frustrated with the free time, something his father would have cherished.

What factors had contributed to the grandson of Al Chanesky suffering a fatal heart attack at age 38? Were they medical or were they sociological problems? Was he the victim of his own habits or had some malignant hand of fate struck him down?

Let's examine briefly the elements leading up to his death.

Number one, the victim smoked. One reason he smoked is because of family tradition. This is not to say that because parents smoke, children will smoke, statistically, however, it has been proven it is much more likely that the children of smokers will smoke. Smoking is one of the leading causes of heart disease. Smoking is certainly not a biological trait passed along from generation to generation; it is a learned characteristic.

Because of no exercise or physical activity in his job, he got fat. The fat accounted for high cholesterol, a large number of low-density lipoproteins, contributing to high blood pressure, elevated triglycerides and excessive blood glucose (from his diet). An EKG would have indicated abnormalities, but the victim avoided doctors and examinations; he knew that he was in poor health. The victim's maximal oxygen consumption wouldn't even be worth considering.

Of the fifteen factors involved, the only one that was not working against him (but that was on the verge of turning on him) was his age. At 38 years old, he should have had a few years left. Unfortunately, the weight of tradition was too heavy and he was doing nothing to help his natural defenses against the onslaught of negative forces in his life.

As we've pointed out, virtually all of these debilitating factors were avoidable. If he'd been born into a different family, or if he'd lived in a healthful environment he would have likely outlived a Galapagos turtle.

His one attempt at exercise—bowling—was merely symbolic. Bowling takes about as much energy as getting up to turn the dial on a television set.

Some simple attention to his own life and a few positive steps, could have made a profound difference in age span for the grandson of Al Chanesky living in the "promised land."

JOINING THE ARMY

By following the story of the Chanesky family, something becomes very apparent. The society that presents the opportunity for developing health problems through laziness also provides the means for overcoming those problems, in the form of leisure time sporting activities.

When Al Chanesky came to the United States, his life, and the life of his wife Erma, revolved almost exclusively around bare existence. He had to work long and hard at his job to earn a living; she had to work diligently to make his pay translate into that bare living. There was little if any time left for anything but the simplest of pleasures: a walk around town on Sunday afternoon, a drink with the boys for Al, some chatting over the rough fences behind the house while hanging up clothes for Erma, an occasional shared moment between work and sleep. Their very lives were an exercise in exercise. They were on the go from before the sun came up until well after it went down. That hardy life provided certain protections, while encouraging other health-related problems. They were toughened against fatigue and developed a certain muscular hardness. But by breaking down their bodies so regularly, they also opened themselves to various diseases that had a way of spreading through towns and cities in those days. Our concern is not, however, with diseases such as scarlet fever or smallpox. It is with heart disease and the role exercise can play in helping to prevent it. We also want to consider exercise for its own sake. And we want to consider the role of lifestyle on one's health and well-being.

It would be difficult, certainly, to picture Al Chanesky and Erma Chanesky going off to a racquetball club for some exercise and then a night out at the juice bar. They didn't need a racquetball club for exercise and wouldn't have had time for one even if such a thing existed.

American society, even at the time Al Chanesky immigrated, was undergoing profound change because of the Industrial Revolution. Jobs of toil were now being done by machines, and people were finding themselves in jobs very much less physically demanding than those performed by their fathers.

Unions were organizing to demand better pay and more humane hours and working conditions. There were more options for those who wished to pursue a higher education, and from there to seek careers unique in the history of their families. More forms of entertainment were being invented and developed. Home appliances were giving the typical housewife more free time. The overall burden of physical labor was being constantly lessened for society, while the availability of more leisure time became more apparent.

It is not so hard to understand why after generations of hard work, most people took the opportunity to rest when the leisure time found its way into their lives. Unfortunately, some later generations were still resting for their grandfathers' exhausting work before them.

In the *Runner's World Indoor Exercise Book*, we referred to the situation as Inertia. A body at rest tends to stay at rest until acted upon by some outside force.

America worked hard to invent leisure time, and then took great advantage of it. People began sitting around watching TV, joining bowling leagues, building rumpus rooms, building barbecue pits in the back yard, going to ballparks to watch professional football and baseball teams, going on picnics, or just taking a Sunday drive in the Oldsmobile.

America, always the leader, was showing the world how to relax, with a vengeance.

Much of the successful relaxing began showing its effects around the belt-line and in the statistics of rising heart disease. Leisure time and less physically strenuous (but often psychologically stressful) jobs, plus learned heredity, combined to create a monster.

But, within the problem lay the solution.

Many Americans who still had vivid memories of their physical shapes when they were ten years younger, began wanting to do something to recapture some of their "better days," before time wiped away even the memory. In unprecedented numbers, they began taking up sports and lifestyles that fit nicely into their available leisure time.

An interesting change began to be noticed. For the first time in generations, the incidence of heart disease in the United States slowed, stopped, and then actually began to reverse itself. Not significantly, certainly, but it was a sign that something positive was happening—a change in priorities. A growing group of Americans was taking charge of their bodies and their lives and they were pointing the way for the rest of the country.

People were running, bicycling, swimming, becoming more physically active; they were joining health spas, doing daily exercise routines, changing their lifestyles. They were finding that it was doing several things for them:

1. Firming and toning muscles and often cutting into unwanted fat.

2. Relieving stress from hectic daily lives.

3. Increasing self-esteem through the reshaping of their bodies and the increased ability to be more active than they'd been in years.

4. Changing habits that they'd felt were ingrained forever, i.e., stopping smoking; it interfered with the ability to exercise well.

5. Enhancing the quality of their lives; instead of watching life go by, they were suddenly part of the passing parade.

In some ways, the exercising movement was a byproduct of what Tom Wolfe had dubbed the "Me Generation" of the 1970s. Instead of trying to solve the problems of the world, as though the United States was the world's policeman, Americans began turning their focus inward, looking closer to home. The attention on "self" in some ways had very chilling and unsettling side effects. Long-running marriages broke up because one or both of the partners decided they wanted a life for themselves, a great deal of selfishness was dished out by a large number of people.

In the end, however, the 1970s may have been more a purging than anything. And all of the consequences were not negative. Certainly the growing awareness that we did not have to sit in front of a TV watching other people move about, take pratfalls, and become people of action was extremely positive. We began to realize that we, too, could become an active part of what was happening in the world around us.

Often frustrated in high school and college by required gym

classes that taught virtually nothing (except sit-ups and pushups) and intimidated by the jocks on the alma mater's teams, we were rapidly finding that there were sports that we could take part in without being judged by our peers. The sports were generally the "individual" sports—running, bicycling, tennis, even bodybuilding. And, for the first time in history, a significant number of us rediscovering participant sports and fitness came from the female side of the country. Long the victims of second-class status within the sports and gymnastics establishments in school, the women of America began taking up sports and fitness with vigor.

Perhaps the whole movement that characterized the late-1970s can be called The Sweat Generation, instead of the Me Generation—at least the subculture of the decade that we are concerned with.

"Sweat of the brow" became a term that was now a brand of participation, a brand of courage of sorts—it marked a person who was taking control of his physical life, who realized that a body, like a car, needs maintenance, or it quickly gets out of tune and eventually ends up on the junk heap. Other cars (and bodies), kept tuned and repaired, some of them twenty and thirty years older, will still ply the highways, getting admiring glances from passing motorists.

A segment of America was interested in reverting, by choice and not by necessity, to the physical activity that marked their ancestors. Although they now worked in an office or in a home replete with timesaving devices, and no longer worked in a steel mill or a coal mine or in a house without appliances, the newly active American grasped good, healthy sweat as the knights of old would have grasped the Grail.

Not everyone who wanted to get involved in the fitness movement had the time or the current fitness to rush right out and enter a marathon in order to assert his new-found awareness of the body.

The emotional damage done by the physical education systems in schools was deep-seated in many instances. Frustrated by school sports that only recognized the burly football player and unsure of their potential, many Americans felt awkward about going outside to exercise. They were shy to show off a body that had not been used in many years, to a country that seemed eminently ready to show off its own physical prowess in the Olympics.

A subculture of the exercise subculture began to form. It had, in many ways, already existed. For years, exercise activists like Jack La Lanne had reached millions in their homes with their exercise programs on television. Exercise was becoming popular but only in the privacy and comfort of the own home.

In some instances, you can't blame them. Who, getting the urge to begin an exercise program in January, wants to go outside when living in Vermont? No one in his right mind, certainly! And why let a good idea ride until spring?

It is very understandable, then, that many people began doing exercises at home. The living room floor or a corner of the bedroom was sufficient space to do a good deal of muscle-toning.

In many instances, the indoor exerciser eventually ventures outside, usually to try out his newly formed body by running on the roads. Others find the indoor exercising sufficient for their needs. Many who exercise most of the time outdoors still spend a certain amount of time indoors doing stretching exercises, yoga, strength training, etc. After a run I find it very relaxint to warm down by stretching on the living room floor or to work out on the Universal weight machine if I'm on a lunchbreak at work.

The manufacturers of indoor exercise equipment soon became aware a new market was building and they began manufacturing at-home versions of their equipment. Some companies, in fact, like SoloFlex, almost redesigned the whole concept of indoor weight exercises by developing a compact and very flexible home gym.

No longer was the person who wanted to exercise indoors faced with the need to join a local spa or gym. A gym, with people as strong as the Incredible Hulk working out on the huge, complex equipment, can be very intimidating. It can also be rather factory-like, and uninviting, despite the mirrors and chrome and uniformed attendants—or perhaps because of them. Additionally, many people who go to gyms and spas spend a half-hour working out and then light up a cigarette!

And, unless you had a million dollars and a large garage, it was impossible to make your own home gym on a level with the local spa or health club. Some of the equipment the gyms use weighs two tons, takes up a tremendous amount of floor space, and looks like a modernized version of something from the bargain basement dungeon at the Spanish Inquisition.

The new equipment is smaller, compact, designed specifically for the home, and can often be integrated with the home atmosphere with little or no problems.

In subsequent chapters we will discuss the major categories of home equipment and examine their design and their use; we will present some typical programs that can be used in conjunction with them and explore two advanced free exercise sequences.

But, assuming that you are interested in learning more about indoor exercising, and that you are anxious to give it a try, let's pause for a moment before getting into those chapters, and examine a very realistic question that has several parts to it. The question involves your getting involved in a vigorous exercise program in the first place.

These are several of the related questions we'll consider:

1. Who should embark on an indoor exercise program?

2. How is it possible to measure your level of fitness before you begin your program?

3. How quickly should you push yourself in your new life as exerciser?

THE QUESTION OF YOUR "STATE OF HEALTH"

Our initial book, the *Runner's World Indoor Exercise Book*, was based on an entry-level format so that it could be used by virtually anyone. It started with the basics, and featured nothing extremely strenuous. By progressing from one chapter to the next, carefully, we could tone up without investing a great deal of time and without a great deal of difficulty and sweat. We made some mild admonitions toward starting slowly, being patient and progressing to the next step carefully. Even a person who was active in school sport is likely to have trouble getting back into training ten years later. A world-class marathoner who becomes injured and has to lay off a mere four weeks, must ease back into training. Our cautions centered on learning to know your own body, to feel how it reacted to your exercise routine and to progress accordingly. It was our feeling that virtually anyone *could* get into an indoor exercise program, and that literally everyone *should*. The stress was on using common sense to dictate progress into more difficult and demanding routines. A 72-year-old woman would want to embark on an indoor exercise program much more slowly and carefully than a 25-year-old woman.

This second book has exercise programs a lot more strenuous and heavy-duty than the initial one, and it subsequently raises the question of just who should embark on a serious, fairly difficult indoor exercise program.

This is a very serious question.

And a very complicated question.

When the running boom began, there was a feeling among runners within the medical profession that you didn't need a medical examination before taking up running, unless you knew you had a serious problem of some sort. Their advice was to take up running very cautiously, certainly, but to skip the examination because in most cases the medical personnel who examined you would advise you against something as strenuous as running. Why? Because they did not understand running and other aerobic sports. They were old-fashioned and they would advise you, if you were beyond college age, to grow up and forget this nonsense about wanting to run. "Why do you want to run, anyway? Didn't you get that out of your system when you were a kid?" they might ask.

The compounding of the problem, warned the runner/doctors, came if you were already running and took an examination to determine your ability to handle sustained exercise. Running causes a sort of advanced fitness in certain systems, and medical examinations are geared toward the sedentary, average American. Certain readings the doctors would be likely to get from an especially fit runner would lead him to interpret it as a sign of degeneration of the body systems, when in actuality it was a sign of fitness.

Dr. George Sheehan, a cardiologist and marathoner from New Jersey, is one of the most eloquent speakers and writers against the traditional physical examination for healthy people. In his excellent book, *Dr. Sheehan on Running*, he has this to say:

"The annual physical examination has been called a useless annual fiasco. I'll drink some Gatorade to that. You can no more give people health than you can give them wisdom. Society can and must guarantee access to educational opportunity and health services, but learning and health are personal responsibilities.

"The main problem with these exams is that the doctor is most concerned with disease. He gives a patient 'a clean bill,' meaning that all tests are normal. He ignores the fact that the patient is actually physically unfit and even a potential candidate for serious disease."

Dr. Sheehan goes on to explain the contribution athletes have made to the medical community:

"Athletes have already done a thorough job of raising the consciousness of physicians interested in sports. They have, among other contributions: (a) established a new normal for man; (b) changed our concept of aging; (c) confirmed the idea of the totality of man, and (d) shifted the emphasis from disease to health.

"Before we discovered that athletes were attaining maximum metabolic, muscular and cardiopulmonary steady states, we were using 'average' individuals as normals. We were, in affect, using life's spectators instead of life's competitors, and were coming up with overweight, out-of-breath subjects testing well below their potential. This can clearly be shown by comparing these psuedo-normals to the athletes in their age group. Their test results are frequently as much as 50 percent below the athletes' performance."

Dr. Sheehan then comments on the problems the athletes faced when they became injured and attempted to find help in a physician's office for what amounted to a byproduct of fitness:

"Would you believe there are people in America in trouble from trying too hard? This information, however implausible, happens to be true. And not a mere handful of dedicated nuts. All over the country, runners, tennis players, football and baseball players, golfers and athletes of all descriptions—pro, amateur, weekend and what have you—are consulting their physicians because of symptoms due to trying too hard.

"The first wave of these patients caught the medical profession by surprise. Doctors are accustomed to seeing man's attempt to maximize himself—but only for ill. They are adjusted to a fat, indolent clientele.

"This gloomy group, however, has become interspersed with an odd bunch who come to the office because of a foot, leg, arm and other pains due to excessive activity. 'It all began,' the patient will say, 'after I started running 100 miles a week.' Or, 'I'd been averaging three hours of tennis a day without trouble when I changed my racket.' Or, 'I wonder if 36 holes three times a week is too much.'

"Medics trained to disease rather than overuse confront these self-maximizers in disbelief, and are unable to give any advice except to cease and desist from such foolishness. This is an unsatisfactory prescription for any athlete, but especially disappointing to one passionate enough to devote the amount of time necessary to develop this type of ailment."

The advice of knowledgeable physicians like Dr. Sheehan was to avoid, like the plague, anyone who would hold you back from courting the injury of fitness.

During that time, Dr. Sheehan and others like him were warning people to avoid physicians of any kind for as long as they could. Their advice was sound. Most physicians were as unfit as their patients, and had no common ground for understanding an athlete's fitness problems.

Credit must be given to some members of the medical profession, however, because after consulting the mounting evidence that exercise could ward off disease, they took up vigorous exercise themselves. They became so caught up in it that they, too, began doing research on exercise. As a result, today we have a new breed of doctor available to those who feel the urge or need to exercise and don't want negative feedback from their personal physician. The doctors are classified under the heading *sportsmedicine*, a classification that can—thank goodness!—extend to your family physician, if he is currently briefed on the benefits of exercise and is an active participant.

The doctors of sportsmedicine will do whatever they can to help a person begin or continue an exercise program. And an exercise program—even a very vigorous one—can be pursued by almost anyone!

Each year at the Honolulu Marathon there is a cardiac division in which people who have suffered from heart disease (whether they be veterans of double bypass surgery or multiple heart attacks) compete at the full twenty-six mile distance. They have been carefully introduced to an exercise program and after about a year their hearts are often healthier and stronger than they were in their youth.

It is an inspiration to hear their stories, how they had allowed themselves to be plagued by disease, sitting around waiting for the next heart attack. Having suffered the extremes of heart disease, they threw all their hopes and drive into an exercise plan. Amazingly, running, bicycling, swimming, vigorous weight-room work, done carefully, gradually and under the direction of their heart specialists, had changed them entirely. They were like new people. They had been given a new lease on life.

Most people enter an exercise program many steps healthier than a heart attack victim. And with the added advantage of having available to them a growing number of talented and expert medical personnel. No longer is the person who contemplates embarking on an exercise program faced with the prospect of getting a lecture from the medical community about the foolishness of such an idea.

In most major metropolitan areas, there are now state-of-the-art facilities available that offer a complete physical test, which is then interpreted by a doctor trained in exercise physiology. He can properly advise you on what steps to take to begin your exercise program. His programs are customized to your current physical condition. On-going consultation is available, as is periodic retesting to monitor progress.

It is time, I feel, that those of you who have been away from strenuous exercise for five years or more seriously consider having such a test to determine your current level of fitness—or lack of fitness. With the facts in front of you, and interpreted by a professional, you can begin a vigorous exercise program with the knowledge that you are not starting too quickly. You can have a scientifically established starting point (complete with a computer printout) and chart your progress in your program.

Although I was also as cynical as Dr. Sheehan about submitting to a physical examination some years ago, my opinion has drastically changed, considering the turnabout in the medical profession that has allowed sportsmedicine specialists to come into their own.

Although I'd been exercising regularly for three years, I decided to go through a complete fitness test, both to see what level I was at (with the idea of trying to ultimately push beyond that level) and to experience firsthand what is involved in a complete fitness test. It was quite a revelation. And quite a change from the old armed forces physical examination where they have you bend over and say "Ah."

What follows is one of the more unforgettable experiences of my life.

THE AGONY AND THE ECSTASY

Outside the window, two secretaries walked through the parking lot, chatted a moment and then parted, one of them lowering herself smoothly into a brown Toyota. The late-afternoon sun was turning the sky from a brilliant blue to a mellow orange. Blocking the lower portion of the window was an electronic cabinet the size of a small dining room hutch. In the upper left portion of the machine an orange number kept changing. It would rise by a dozen numbers, pause, and then drop and settle at a slightly higher level temporarily. At the moment it was at 110, about to take another jump.

"You'll go to stage four in about five seconds," George M.

Oehlsen, the bearded and nattily mustachioed laboratory director intoned solemnly. "This will be the stage in which you can move from fast walking to slow jogging." Before he finished speaking, there was a barely audible click, and then the computer in front of me sent the treadmill's speed up a notch and raised its angle another 2 percent.

Carrying a 6-oz. plastic fluid bottle on a run throws off my balance and stride, but the treadmill test at the S.M.A.R.T. (Sports Medicine Athletic Rehabilitation & Training) Clinic in Cupertino, California was making matters much worse. You know the picture: white-coated technicians standing around with clipboards watching a runner chug along on a moving belt, wires running from a dozen contact points on his body, while his head, with a mask and hose attached to it, looks like something from *"20,000 Leagues Under the Sea."* Looking at the picture and thinking about it is the easy part. Trying to run under such conditions is a completely different matter. It gives you a new appreciation of why a 1970 fully equipped Cadillac needed a 450-plus cubic inch engine to reach the same speeds as a 1970 Triumph TR-6, which featured an engine 25 percent the Caddy's size. Make the Caddy engine handle power steering, air conditioning, power windows, power seats, power brakes, anti-pollution equipment, and you have a car struggling uphill while it's idling at a stop light.

The analogy was going through my mind as I "tried" to run. A black box strapped to my back directly over my right buttock had a dozen lines running from it to patches taped on my chest and sides which were taking electronic "pictures" of my heart. It struggled, like the Caddy's gas pump, to meet the regularly increasing demands of a body in distress. The wires coming out the other end of the black box fed into the compact little computer in the cabinet against the wall. If my heart so much as thought ill will against me during the ordeal, the machine picked it up and recorded it for all time.

Rod Wight, a cardiac nurse, stood next to my right elbow taking my blood pressure readings while the machine in front of me recorded my pulse rate from an instrument he'd placed against my inner arm, right next to the ubiquitous blood pressure wrap. Several times during each three-minute stage, Wight would pump up the wrap, take my blood pressure, and call it out to George, who would write it down on the tape coming out of the machine.

They had also put a frame around my head that held a plastic

Just How Fit is Fit? (or, Survival of the Fittest) 27

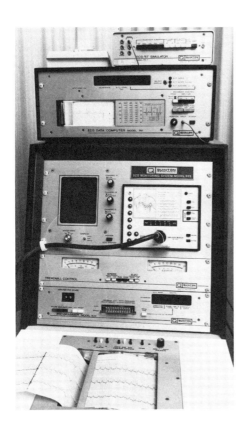

The wonderful world of electronics has had a profound effect upon the medical and health establishment by providing the means for carefully monitoring all the major body systems (left) without the hardware taking up a three-story building. Pictured is the Quinton Instruments ECG monitoring System model 633, a compact unit that has made modern fitness testing centers practical and profitable. Before the treadmill testing is conducted, George Oehlsen hooks up the author to the monitoring machinery, and takes a preliminary blood pressure reading, which in this case was high due to the author's anticipation of the testing.

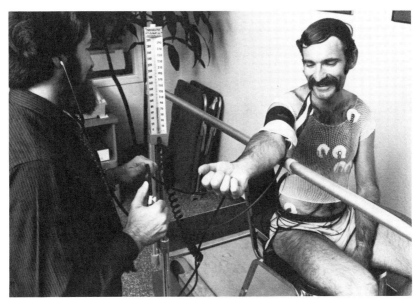

28 JUST HOW FIT IS FIT? (OR, SURVIVAL OF THE FITTEST)

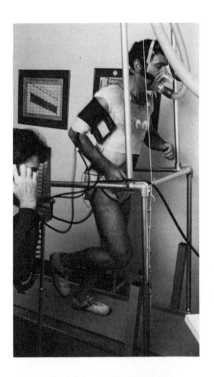

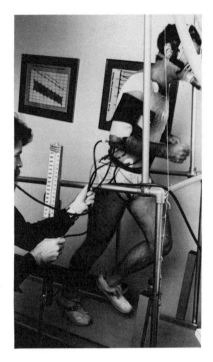

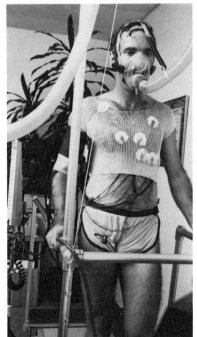

The test begins with a walking pace, and every three minutes, the pace is picked up, and the angle of attack is raised. George (upper left) takes periodic blood pressure readings, while the monitoring equipment keeps track of other vital signs. As the speed of the belt increases and the angle of attack rises, the author's effort skyrockets (upper right), the wires and hook-ups becoming a burden. Having given the "I give up!" signal (keft), the author drops back to a walking pace.

mask over my nose and mouth. A plastic hose about two inches in diameter ran from the front of the mask to a machine on one of the cabinet's shelves. The mask-hose attachment collected all the gases I exhaled and all the air I inhaled also came through the hose; on the shelf there were measuring devices, which registered the volume of air I breathed in and blew out. Earlier I had determined which one did which, because even without wearing my glasses, the read-out numbers were large enough that I could see their orange figures jump rapidly when I blew out or sucked in air. When I started this trial I had found the pulse rate number and the exhale/inhale numbers and enjoyed watching them change by blowing little bursts of air through the hose. The exhale numbers would flick up by twenty or twenty-five points each breath. At the time it seemed fascinating that every puff of air was being followed so closely; but as the treadmill began to demand more from me, I began to resent its knowing so accurately that it was getting its pound of flesh.

Considering my condition, I didn't feel things were going well.

Three weeks previous, an old injury had reoccurred. Connecting tissue between the top of the Achilles tendon and the bottom of the calf muscle on the right leg, which had originally been torn several years before in a motorcycling accident, had apparently torn again. Training had dropped from an off-season 45 miles per week to a mere 15 miles per week. Also, my right arm swings more vigorously than my left when I run, but it was impeded here by the blood pressure wrap. I had to run with my elbows awkwardly tucked against my sides. Further, I have a habit of swinging my elbows out toward my sides, which compensates the tendency of my legs to "roll" around the outside of my hips when going uphill, rather than pumping from directly under my body. This motion was restricted by the safety rails on the sides of the treadmill. To make matters worse, because my head was pulled up by the straps and hoses, I could not see the treadmill running surface and fought a constant sensation of being on the verge of falling. I felt like Orson Welles trying to run stadium steps while blindfolded and wearing a straightjacket. "It's sure easy to see he's a runner," Rod said to George. "You can barely hear his feet striking the belt." But I could clearly hear each awkward impact; and even if I couldn't have heard it, I'd have thought I did from the dull pains shooting up from my right calf and Achilles as the angle of treadmill's running surface got steeper. I wondered if the only test subjects they'd used previously had been three-legged elephants.

Rod wasn't accustomed to seeing subjects with my health. He had spent seven years in an intensive and coronary care unit, administering to seriously ill people, 60-70 percent of whom he felt wouldn't be there if they'd payed attention to exercise and diet. "Preventive health is the key to better health and lower overall medical costs," he'd said. "With proper diet and adequate exercise the average person in this country can improve his overall health profile significantly." Perhaps he was experiencing *deja vu*; perhaps he thought he was hearing hopeful footsteps from a person formerly believed to be half-dead.

I blew a long breath out and watched the orange numbers flick upward, upward. I gazed at the pulse rate indicator, wondering how high it would go when we moved into stage five. I gazed out the window and there was nobody in the parking lot. Just a deepening orange from the setting sun. I tried to think about a peaceful beach, but it didn't work. The pulse rate indicator continued to climb....

Runners and other athletes have always been curious about how their bodies work, and how well they are working at any set time in their training process. They have traditionally gauged their training by intuition, by how they felt, by how long it took to recover from a prescribed workout. A growing list of scientists equally interested in knowing what makes us tick have paralleled the growth of sports and athletes in the United States. They are investigating the limits of man's endurance, human biomechanics and physiology, and precisely measuring man's struggle to push back his perceived limits. How do genes affect an athlete's performance? How much training is too much? Can variations in training improve an athlete's oxygen uptake capacity? What chemical changes come into play during heavy training? Why do muscles tire? How does the cardiovascular system of a distance runner differ from that of a two-pack-a-day cigarette smoker who never exercises?

After some initial suspicion and mistrust, the well-trained athletes and the scientists began comparing notes. The athletes offered themselves as guinea pigs so that more could be learned about the well-trained body. Advances in the electronics and telemetry industries (fostered by the space program) allowed for machines and instruments that could monitor the athletes' bodies with great accuracy. Long-distance runners and bicycle racers became the

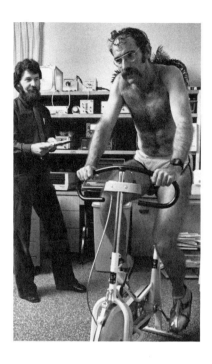

One of the tests involved in the complete fitness evaluation involves strength and speed. An exercise cycle is used. A resistance setting is made, and then the subject climbs aboard and tries to pump as fast as possible for a minute. Pacing is all important, or else your legs turn to lead in the final 15 seconds.

scientists' favorite subjects. "They don't seem to mind pain and discomfort," Dr. David Costill a leading authority in the field and head of Ball State University's biomechanics laboratory once said. "Sprinters, boxers, football players—they're all difficult to work with. But runners and cyclists seem to thrive on being tested, no matter what they have to pay in discomfort."

Just as the scientific community began gearing up for increased experimentation, the exercise boom struck with a gasp for breath that was heard round the world. Suddenly the testing procedures being developed to probe the inner workings of a few select athletic guinea pigs could now be used in a myriad of ways on a new army of neo-athletes. They could find out if a sedentary 55-year-old was safe to start a vigorous cycling program without harming his heart, lungs and muscles. They could carefully monitor heart attack victims who were attempting to fight their way back to health on an exercise program. They could help experts customize exercise programs. And they could give the curious exerciser an accurate picture of his physical shape. In less than eight hours of testing time, you can be supplied with more information about yourself than you would know what to do with. In its way, the Age of Testing had arrived.

Where before, a few select, colleges had amassed testing equipment and know-how, with funding from government grants and university endowments, testing facilities in the private sector were sprouting up, ready to handle the increasing number of runners, bicyclists, tennis players and swimmers who would be willing to pay for their own testing.

Today every major metropolitan area in the country boasts a sophisticated diagnostic testing facility for the human machine. They are growing at a rate not dissimilar to the spread of automobile garages following the introduction of the horseless carriage. It would be impossible to survey all of them; it would also be very confusing, because although all of these testing facilities give essentially the same tests, their equipment and techniques may be entirely different.

Because of its proximity to my office and because of some unique features, I chose the S.M.A.R.T. Clinic in Cupertino, California, a facility that offers testing, training and rehabilitation. Founded in 1975 by two orthopedic surgeons, a professional football player and a physical therapist, the facility was designed to offer sophisticated training for full-time athletes on both a collegiate and professional level, as well as rehabilitation facilities.

Six months after its opening, George Oehlsen, who has a M.A. in human performance and exercise physiology, joined the clinic to set up a testing wing. The testing was to benefit the hard-core athlete, for whom the clinic was originally founded, but it was also to be made available to the non-athlete. Eventually the professional football player and the physical therapist sold out to the two orthopedic surgeons, and the clinic began moving in a slightly different direction. It continued to offer an extensive Nautilus-based training facility and a rehabilitation facility for the college and professional athlete, and began placing an equal emphasis on complete physical testing of corporate executives, weekend athletes, and plain-old walking-around folks.

George's philosophy was quite simple and straightforward: "Educating the public to gain a better understanding of the disease process would help to lower the incidence of disease in the United States. By disease I mean heart disease. And heart disease primarily results from two of about a dozen factors, excessive caloric and fat intake. It's no longer a 'lifestyle' disease, but a 'deathstyle' disease, because people are killing themselves. Quality of life should be more important than quantity of life, and luckily many people are coming around to learn what they can do to repair the damage they've done to themselves over the years."

After the testing, a complete exercise and dietary program can be prescribed for a client, and much of the exercise can be accomplished on the equipment at the facility. A unique approach was instigated when George, in setting up the procedures, played everything off a small, but sophisticated computer. ("We have an advantage," George said, "in that we live in the back yard of the largest electronics complex in the world.") When all the testing is finished, from flexibility to dietary, treadmill to skin-fold, and the results are fed into the computer, a 35-page "book" on the person being tested is delivered. The "book" is then bound and the person's name is printed in gold on the front. The person's physical biography for that point in his life is explained in an eminently personalized style.

The cost of the entire evaluation, which covers 10 categories, including chest X-ray and medical examination by a doctor, is $360. Without the chest X-ray and doctor's examination the price drops to $280. (If you are covered by standard medical insurance, and the testing and evaluation is prescribed by a physician, the insurance usually pays 80 percent of the cost.)

S.M.A.R.T.'s clients currently range from nine to sixty-five years of age. Their occupations are as varied as the typical American public: businessmen, homemakers, professional athletes, carpenters, a few world-record holders, insurance salesmen.

The S.M.A.R.T. philosophy for undergoing the tests boils down to "A fit body is a happy body." And their exercise prescription following the testing evaluation, depending on the sport you wish to advance in, sends you outside for aerobic exercising more than it advises exercising with formal bodybuilding equipment. Running, bicycling, swimming and stretching exercises are integral parts of their exercise suggestions.

They will test almost anyone, although if testing is contraindicated by medical history, the tests will be modified to accommodate you. George Oehlsen says that he's saving all the test results on the computer, and that ultimately they will be compared to averages of others tested as well as the "average" American population.

If you've ever watched an afternoon sky, you've seen its early, subtle changes begin to accelerate as the sun drops toward the horizon. The colors become rich and full as night rushes forward.

I had plenty of time to take in the changing hues through the lab's window. The orange colors were beginning to darken into rust and their changes, I suspected, were happening over a matter of hours. Actually, only seconds were passing.

I felt that I should have moved from stage four into stage five by now, but nothing was happening around me to indicate a change. The treadmill continued to whir and my breathing attempted to stabilize, but fell just short as George stood over the paper printout marking down numbers. Rod occasionally pumped up the blood pressure indicator and gave him a reading. Perspiration began trickling down my sides from my armpits despite the presence of a cooling fan, and it made my mustache slick, causing the face mask to slip. I reached up with my left hand to readjust it and tried to encourage my legs to smooth out, but there were too many factors working against them. My style stayed ragged. I wished for a wall clock in front of me, over the window, so I could see how much time was left for stage four. George would tell me when I was about to enter the next stage, but only some five seconds in advance.

Squinting my eyes until they closed, I tried to blot out the monotony of the effort. It didn't work. I opened them just in time to see the hose in front of my face disconnect from my face mask. "Just keep running," George said. "We'll take care of it." He moved over, reached up and reattached the hose. For a moment, whether real or imagined, I'd felt a mite revived by room air being sucked into my lungs, because it wasn't going the long route through the machinery.

I was just beginning to notice a tightness in my legs and once again question the wisdom of going through with this thing when George's voice broke in: "Stage five coming up in five seconds." I felt myself tensing for the treadmill acceleration and the raising of the angle of attack by two degrees more. I called myself a fool but it was lost in a gasp for more air. Night couldn't fall soon enough to suit me.

Two days before, in the early morning, I'd gone to the clinic, a modern, spacious building dominated by a graphic symbol of a highly-musculatured and stylized male with a Nautilus worked into his right hip. The first order of business was to fill out a medical history, followed by a dietary form, which asked for a typical weekday's ingestion of food, and a typical weekend day's ingestion, the logic being that your eating habits often change when the weekend comes and you go off your rather regimented weekday routine. It is surprising how difficult it is to remember *exactly* and *completely* what you ate in the past twenty-four hours. The form featured worksheets at the back where your meals could be broken down by food and amount and given a value that would mysteriously translate itself into calories taken in, complete with a percentage of carbohydrates, fats and proteins. There were several blank boxes at the end where "one $1.14 bag of Cheetos" found its home. The ubiquitous combination pizza spread itself all over the worksheets with its bell peppers, pepperoni, mushrooms, black olives, cheeses, cashews (We eat differently in California than the rest of the world), ham, pineapple, etc., to appropriate boxes.

Height and weight were taken, blood drawn, strength tested in

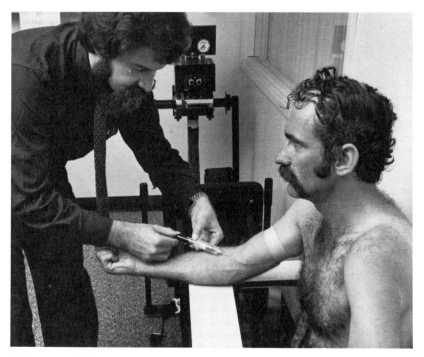

Perhaps one of the most important and comprehensive tests is the blood test. Sophisticated lab techniques make it possible to read an incredible amount of information from a small sampling of blood. Without asking, the author feels that George is a guy who finds Halloween his favorite holiday.

my arms and legs by using the sophisticated Cybex machines, and in my stomach by sixty seconds of sit-ups. Speed and agility were tested by a race end to end on a wrestling mat while picking up

JUST HOW FIT IS FIT? (OR, SURVIVAL OF THE FITTEST)

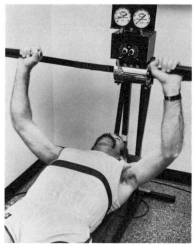

The Cybex machines measure strength and power.

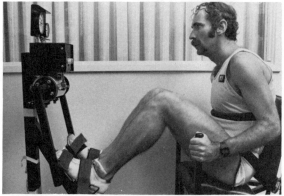

Force is exerted quickly against the machine.

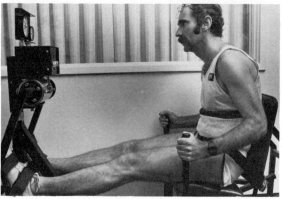

The machine's resistance comes from a fluid-filled cylinder.

Just How Fit is Fit? (or, Survival of the Fittest) 37

and dropping blackboard erasers; flexibility limitations were tested by forcing my body to stretch to its limits in a variety of directions; a test of lung capacity was made; a skin-fold test for body fat was done; evaluation of musculo-skeletal balance was made, and finally, the ultimate indignity: dunking as punishment for witchcraft.

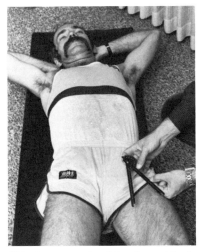

This is a test to determine subject's range of motion.

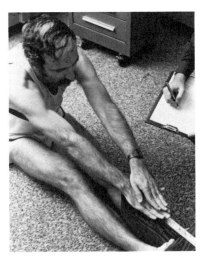

The author's flexibility is two points behind a dry twig.

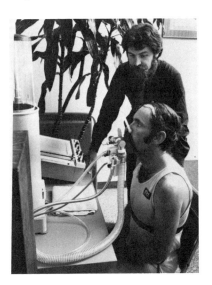

The subject's lung capacity is tested and measured and is later also used in creating an accurate measurement in the water displacement testing for fat content. The challenge of this test is trying to expel the maximum amount of air in the lungs and to hold it until a measurement is made; there is residual air left in the lungs, but the human mind reads this test as an earthside approximation of what it would feel like to step outside an orbiting spacecraft while wearing only swimming trunks.

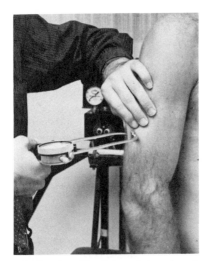 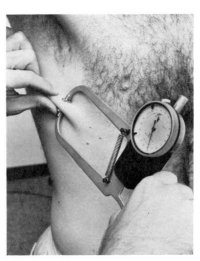

Fat, fat, fat. The bane of America, is being measured.

The calipers are not a totally accurate method, but come close.

Most people are familiar with the sophisticated method of measuring body fat by immersion in water. In theory, the body (if properly weighed down) will displace a certain amount of water, while the body's fat, which is lighter than water, will attempt to bring the body to the surface. (An extension of the childhood realization that the fatter kids in your class always seemed to be able to float better.) Measurements must be made, however, so the victim is placed into a chair, not too unlike those used to dunk witches in colonial Salem; the chair is attached to a scale in the ceiling. Before getting into the chair, the person straps on a weight belt like skin divers use. The water, so as not to shock the person with a bad heart, is kept very warm; consequently, to retard the growth of algae, the chlorine level is kept two points below lethal.

The process for the immersion test is to have the testee get into the chair, exhale every possible cubic inch of air in his lungs (It is physically impossible to exhaust all air in his lungs, but the lung capacity test done previously gives a good measure of the testee's parameters.), and then submerge, hanging relaxed and limp in the chair for ten seconds. In order to get a fair test, the process must be repeated five times.

Sounds easy—if you're a fish that likes chlorine. Considering that every time I've gone into fresh water and tried to float I've dropped like a rock to the bottom, the test seemed easy. In self-defense I'd spent much of my childhood tadpoling it around the

Just How Fit is Fit? (or, Survival of the Fittest) 39

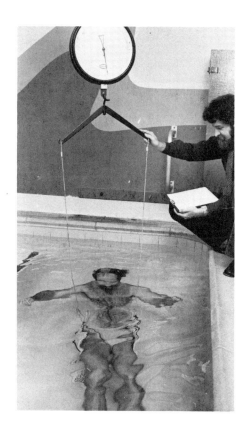

This is more like it. A swim in warm water. Actually, this was worst part of the entire testing, involving going underwater, expelling all the air in the lungs, and then resting there calmly as your life rushes past in front of your eyes. Snorkels are not allowed.

bottom of pools and creeks wearing a facemask and flippers, staying away from the surface.

Unfortunately, it is completely different when you go under water with no air and then try to calmly remain submerged for ten seconds, thinking you're going to die. They say that death by drowning is very peaceful and calm, but they haven't taken the time to interview drowning victims to get their view.

The first time under I exhaled all the air I could find in my lungs, was sumberged and then tried to remain calm while counting to ten, as I was told to do. On about four, something tickled my throat and I reacted by trying to pull some air in through my nose. What I got was a nose and throat full of chlorine-saturated water, which brought on a cough reaction that I manfully suppressed until I rushed my count to ten, breaking the surface like a humpback whale trying to fly.

After a great deal of splashing and sputtering—and breathing—we did it again, and again, and again, and again. Near-drowning is a good note on which to end the first day's sessions. It serves to warn the unwary of the capacities for discomfort available on Treadmill Day.

The face mask seemed to be confining my ability to breathe, besides the plain psychological fact that it was something totally unnatural and felt like a gag. The treadmill's angle of attack was taking its toll on my Achilles tendons. In stage five, I was struggling up an 18 percent grade at 4.75 mph. The grade was stretching my tendons beyond the point of comfort into the world of pain. The connecting tissue on the right leg began to protest but the complaints were being drowned in a backwash of sensations that made individual pains, discomforts and observations blend into a sort of phrenetic stew. *"I should have done some hill training,"* I muttered to myself as I tried to focus on something, anything. I found that the orange, digital numbers that had been a comfort now an annoyance—a reminder that someone else knew, down to the segmented gasp for air, how distressed I was becoming.

My distress began to swirl around me, a caldron of uncooked and tasteless raw nerves. Momentarily closing my eyes, trying to remove myself from it, I sensed a heightening paranoia about falling off the end of the treadmill. I snapped my eyes open again. Although I was pulling in enough breath to fan a locomotive's fire, and felt as though there was one flaming furiously in my lungs, I seemed to be two quarts in arrears for each breath. Through the distress and confusion I began to discern a guaranteed breaking point. My thighs were tightening, and becoming like dead weight. They were unused to this. I tried to hyperventilate, hoping to catch up on some oxygen debt and stave off the lactic acid build-up, but I knew it was all happening too fast.

I wanted a clock on the wall telling me how many minutes I had to go to reach stage six, but there was no clock and minutes had turned into eternities. I tried desperately to hold on, but knew that I was slipping. "Don't try to beat the machine," they'd said, "because it can't be done." What instructions, I wondered, did they give to the machine before it got hold of a person? "Don't worry about him beating you, Mr. Treadmill, you've got all the aces..."

The second session started by meeting Dr. Michael Marenchic, who had examined my medical history and dietary habit based on the forms I filled out in the first session. He discussed parts of the forms, asked for details on my childhood diseases and wanted more information on my family's history of heart disease, ulcers and back problems. He also asked for amplification of certain eating patterns, trying to make sure that I'd put down everything I'd eaten on an average day.

He already had the results of my blood tests and remarked on them casually enough to indicate that I was at least safe in that regard. I posessed sufficient blood to keep myself going through the upcoming treadmill test, and I had no abnormalities, that couldn't be explained by my physical activity anyway.

Following some further discussion of the dietary forms and the treadmill test, Dr. Marenchic performed a physical examination; it was somewhere between an Army physical and a NASA astronaut's weekly physical in thoroughness.

"Just try to relax during the treadmill test, as though you were going out on your daily run," he said.

He led me to the treadmill room where George Oehlsen was waiting, an amused smile on his face. After removing my shirt, I was asked to climb up on the treadmill and sit down on a chair that was sitting on the belt. They began attaching their wires and hoses and I began considering the treadmill as some mechanical bull that I was about to challenge. Despite the fact that I knew I couldn't beat it, I could feel the competitive juices beginning to flow. By the time they had everything hooked up and were monitoring me, my blood pressure was 140/96. At this level it was registering a hypertension of sorts—tension to get on with the test. Once the treadmill test began, my blood pressure came down—much the same situation a runner undergoes trying to catch butterflies in his stomach before the race starts. In this case, the starter's gun was a simple sentence as they pushed the buttons to start the test: "Let's get started." For the moment, at least, their use of the term "Let's" felt very comforting; it was as though they would be on the belt with me.

Legend has it that someone once went to stage eight on the treadmill test. Although George Oehlsen admitted to never having met the guy, he did know men, however, who'd gone to stage seven. The machine was capable of going to stage ten, a point at which Superman begins to develop shinsplints. I knew I was more than halfway through stage five, but had absolutely no idea how far beyond halfway. Each successive stage, although a uniform three minutes, seemed to push through to a new time warp, making logical a sense of time more and more meaningless. A fanciful picture my mind had created floated in front of my eyes, pretty much like what Dorothy saw from her bedroom window as her house whirled up toward Oz—the mean old witch floating in air on her bicycle. But my vision was of the legendary Iron Man who had gone to stage eight on the treadmill. He had a barrel chest (in order to suck in the needed oxygen), narrow hips, short and mightily muscled legs with claws instead of toes (enabling him to run up the ever-increasing angle of the treadmill surface), huge arms that he pumped vigorously and that, when the going got rough, just ripped the blood pressure strap right off his arm so that he wouldn't be encumbered by it. He was beetle-browed, had cast-iron teeth, was covered with a thick mat of dung-colored fur, and wore a red cape featuring an "I" beam bursting out of a yellow triangle. He looked exactly like the older brother of a girl I dated in college.

He was a runner, to whom the word "wall" merely meant something to be knocked down.

I tried to encourage him to stay longer than the fleeting moment he occupied my vision, but he had other worlds to conquer and had to leave me to my physical troubles. My right calf was becoming increasingly sore and weak, and through the assault of sensations, my concern for it predominated. I was sucking in air at a frantic, out-of-control rate, but still could not get enough; I was perspiring freely; my running style, which had never smoothed, was deterioriating rapidly. I felt like I was running underwater. My thighs, which develop with hill training and bicycle racing, were tightening up and becoming weak. I wanted to make it to stage six but had no idea how long I had to go to make it. By pushing into exhaustion, if there were only a handful of seconds to go, I could do it—but I had no idea whether I had five seconds or fifty seconds to go.

I reached my hands out to the bar in front of me and grasped it, the prearranged signal that I wanted to stop. They cautioned me to keep going while they slowed the machine, so they could monitor my vital signs to make sure I wasn't going to drop dead on them. The time it took my body to return to a resting state would also be an additional indicator of my fitness—or lack of it.

The machine slowed gradually, and they began removing apparatus from me: first the breathing mask and hose, a little later the blood pressure arm wrap, and finally, they stopped the belt and had me sit down so they could remove the waist belt holding the collector for the dozen wires going to locations on my chest. "Now comes the worst part," Rod Wight said as he guided me off the treadmill to the floor. "We've got to pull the leads off your skin. I hope we shaved off most of the hair under them."

I laughed uneasily, feeling somewhat depressed now that I was off the machine. My legs were still a bit weak but the inevitable conviction that *"You could have gone farther if you'd have pushed it just a little more"* was sinking in. My right calf was my only ally in trying to convince myself that I had done the right thing by stopping. "How much farther did I have to go to reach stage six?" I asked George.

"There were 12 seconds left in stage five," he said.

"It figures," I muttered to myself as Rod yanked off the first lead.

The third visit, which can come as soon as two days following the treadmill test, is a sort of combination graduation and reading of the will.

The visit consists of an hour session with George Oehlsen, in which he presents the book, on which your name is embossed. The book contains ten chapters:

1. Medical profile
2. Nutritional analysis
3. Sports readiness analysis
4. Coronary risk factor profile
5. Cardiovascular fitness profile
6. Body composition
7. Musculo-skeletal evaluation
8. Flexibility
9. Blood chemistry
10. Exercise prescription

The medical profile comes from a combination of the client's medical history as written on the form provided during the first visit and information gleaned from the discussion with the physician. The opening page on medical history explains the relationship that can exist between good health and regular exercise. It stresses the philosophy of prevention over the traditional treatment of symptoms of ill-health.

The next page is the summary of data, which includes anthropometric, cardiovascular and blood chemistry results.

Under anthropometric, your weight is given in kilograms and in pounds, height in centimeters, percentage of body fat and the corresponding lean mass, in kilograms, which is determined by dividing your body fat percentage into your total weight and then subtracting the fat from the total to get lean mass, or the weight of everything in your body, from bones to bowels, that isn't fat. I stopped in my tracks here. My body fat, as measured on the immersion test, was 18.86 percent! In a test of elite runners performed in 1975 at the Aerobics Institute in Dallas, it was found that elite marathoners had an average fat percentage of 4.3, elite middle-distance runners 5.0, good runners 6.1 and average young men 13.4. Active males my own age come in at 18.31 percent. (The average male adds about ½ percent body fat per year after age 20.) Although nearly four years before I'd weighed 207, I was down to 169 after a winter of limited running. I could only conclude that there was a lot of leftover fat floating around in my body. Or that I hadn't blown out nearly enough air when I went under water in the pool. My skin-fold test showed 13.86 percent body fat. I indicated that perhaps I should go on a diet real soon. George indicated otherwise. "When you diet, you lose weight you won't want to; nearly three-quarters of what you lose in dieting is weight in muscles. What you need is a more thorough exercise program," he said. I wondered where I'd get the time for that.

Under cardiovascular, my blood pressure (140/96) had been high as I was prepared for the treadmill test, but that was written off to anticipation, because it dropped as soon as I began the test. My work time on the test had been 14.8 minutes, and I'd been in stage five. My VO_2 max was 66, which was low when compared to the Dallas test of elite athletes. The highest recording in that test was by the late Steve Prefontaine, who came in at 84.4; Frank Shorter's was 71.3. Good runners are figured to be 69.2, while untrained, lean men are 54.2. VO_2 max is the measurement of your ability to make effective use of oxygen under maximum workload; in other words, how good is your oxygen delivery system to your muscles when they really need the oxygen to function? You are somewhat limited in your VO_2 max by nature; by proper training and exercise, however, you can improve it to a limited extent. In other words, if you take the test the week before your marathon personal record, you are going to have a higher score than you would if you took it during a slow training period three months later.

The results are computed to come up with a maximum mets number, which is an easily understood measurement of oxygen uptake stripped of all the scientific overtones. The computerized programs that the S.M.A.R.T. Clinic uses are keyed to your number of mets. A person very much out of shape and perhaps on the verge of collapse would come in at one met, and all progressive exercise programs would be based on that one met as a starting point. Mine came in at nineteen, which would cause some humorous havoc with my suggested exercise program later in the S.M.A.R.T.

My heart rate when I'd given in to the treadmill was 187; 90 percent of that is 175 and 60 percent is 140. Those numbers are valuable because some of the exercises suggested later call for performances at certain percentages of maximum heart rate. To arrive at those percentages, the maximum heart rate had to be learned. It seemed to me, more and more, that I was dogging it on the treadmill test. A maximum heart rate of 187 didn't seem all that high.

The blood chemistry gives five readings: cholesterol (in my case 253, quite high), high-density lipoproteins (HDL) (71, again, quite high, but in this case a good sign, since HDL scrubs the artery walls of plaque), low-density lipoproteins (LDL) (171, relatively high, but held in control by my HDL level), triglycerides (57) and glucose (101). Blood chemistry would be explained later in the book.

The next page explains body fat and how misleading body weight can be when considered against typical wall charts. The ideal weight, according to the book, is based on three criteria: a weight consistent with good health, a weight consistent with your idea of fashion, and a weight that allows you to perform the physical tasks that you want to perform. Your body fat level is charted relative to other age groups and lifestyles.

There is also a chart that predicts how much weight you would have to lose in order to bring your body fat percentages down to limits you might find more pleasant.

The matter of VO_2 max is dealt with next. An explanation of the procedure used to measure VO_2 max is given, and how the result is used to help evaluate your exercise capabilities at this point. There is also information on the electrocardiogram that monitored me during the test; a copy of those results is kept at the lab for comparison purposes in case you come back for retesting, or for your physician's use, if needed. At the bottom of the page a chart gives low, poor, fair, good and high levels of VO_2 max for both sexes and various age groups. At 66, I was well above the target level for males a decade younger.

The next two pages are graphs taken from the treadmill test. The first matches the ventilation and the heart rate, showing curved lines heading toward each other until they intersect, which indicates where the subject reaches his anaerobic threshold. Mine didn't quite meet; I must have had something left. The second graph was a recording of the VO_2 and heart rate.

The following two pages are a complete blood chemistry breakdown and comparison between average values and your own. Pages of explanations of what the readings mean follow. The blood test checks sixteen factors, including the three types of lipoproteins in your blood. Lipoproteins can tell you more about yourself than the simple cholesterol reading. Recent research has indicated that although low-and very low-density lipoproteins are negative factors (that contribute to plaque developing along the walls of the arteries), high-density lipoproteins scrub the LDL off the walls of the arteries. HDL levels can be increased by taking up aerobic exercise and by consuming moderate amounts of alcohol, among other things; they can be retarded by smoking, or by inhaling someone else's smoke.

Fluid levels in the blood are also new and interesting readings. Blood is a fluid, or medium in which nutrients and oxygen are transported to the body's cells. You probably learned when you were children about white blood cells (which fight infection) and red blood cells (which are like serving trays that whizz around the body delivering food to the cells and taking back empty plates and bowls to be washed or disposed of). The normal level of white blood cells for someone my age (35) is between 4.8 and 10.8; I have 4.5. The average for red blood cells is 4.6 to 6.2; mine is 4.87. Two other factors in considering blood make-up are hemoglobin and hematocrit; for the former, the average is 14 to 18 and for the latter, the average is 42 to 52; my values were 14.9 and 43.6. "All of them are on the low end," I said. "Am I in trouble?"

"Not exactly," George reassured me. "If you were not doing aerobic training we might worry about you, except that your mean cell and mean corpuscular hemoglobin concentrations are well up. What your readings indicate is that your body has adapted to your training by storing more fluids in your blood system. During an 18-miler, then, your body will be fed some fluids directly from your bloodstream, whereas a non-exercising person would not have the stored fluids to call upon. If we were to take another blood sample after an 18-miler on a warm day, we'd find that your white blood cell, red blood cell, hemoglobin and hematocrit levels would be at a normal level because your blood would have given up the extra fluid. A day later, however, your body would have restored that fluid to your blood, making itself ready for the next long effort."

"Like a camel," I said.

"Precisely."

"But I still don't like running in the heat," I concluded.

We then discussed the nutritional analysis. Because of its flagrant disregard of the typical meat and potatoes, three-meals-a-day philosophy, I'll mention it only briefly. A well-balanced diet calls for 50 percent carbohydrates (fuel), 15 percent protein (muscle-building materials) and 35 percent fat. People who exercise are advised to decrease their fat intake and elevate their carbohydrate consumption. My diet analysis showed that on typical days, I was consuming less calories than I should for my workload. I agreed with these results, because I was attempting to lose a few pounds before starting my spring training routine.

Much of my diet consists of pizza, which, I have theorized, contains virtually every nutrient you need, if you order the deluxe. George confirmed, by the way, that a deluxe pizza provides a well-rounded meal, as long as you go easy on the meat (which has a high fat content); the pizza crust contains carbohydrates; the cheese contains calcium, and the tomato sauce, bell peppers, mushrooms, black olives, tomato slices, onions, etc., provide minerals and vitamins.

We next discussed my heart attack risk profile. The following factors are considered: systolic blood pressure, diastolic blood pressure, cigarette smoking, cholesterol, LDL/HDL, cholesterol/HDL, triglycerides, blood glucose, percentage body fat, stress-tension index, amount of physical activity, maximal oxygen consumption, S-T index (referring to heart muscle efficiency), family history of heart disease, and age. Most factors are products of family history and inherited social habits, as I discussed earlier, in the example of Al Chanesky and offspring.

The scale ranges from very low, low, moderate, high, to very high. My risk factor was low. Five factors involved the computer program. My systolic blood pressure and diastolic blood pressure were taken as I was being strapped up for the stress test. The anticipation of going against the machine had elevated my blood pressure but once on the machine and into the test, my blood pressure had dropped. Oehlsen discounted these two factors because of my nervousness.

My cholesterol level was high, but we decided that it was offset by my high level of high density lipoproteins.

My glucose level was also high (101 when it should have been less than 90), but that could be controlled with diet, weight control and exercise. One cause for the high reading may have been due to my eating a lot of sweets. Much of the extra energy is burned when I exercise.

Because of the constant pressure I face in meeting deadlines on a magazine, there is little I can do to escape some heavy stress. One way I deal with it is to accept the stress, not fight it, and turn at least some of the stress into a positive factor. Regular exercise is also an excellent reducer of the negative effects of stress.

The five sports I'd picked from the list (distance running, marathon, bicycling, cross-country skiing and downhill skiing) were analyzed based on strength, speed and flexibility tests I'd taken. The results indicated where I'd need development. For example, in the marathon, I need more strength in order to get through the latter miles. The Cybex machine indicated I had plenty of leg strength but my stomach muscles were weak. Also covered was muscular endurance, cardiovascular efficiency, upper body strength, lower body strength, upper body flexibility, lower body flexibility, speed and agility. The book also contained exercises that would improve my performance in each of those areas, and also gave a prescription for strengthening exercises.

The book finishes with an endurance exercise program based on running and bicycling. This is where the matter of "mets," which I discussed earlier, comes in. After a quick examination of the charts and a nervous gulp, I discovered that, should I manage to follow the program through to its conclusion, World-class milers Steve Ovett and Sebastian Coe were in danger of being defeated.

The program is based on progressively more difficult workloads, keyed to a percentage of maximum heart rate. Your maximum heart rate is recorded during the treadmill test; mine had been a paltry 187, due in part to my legs giving out before other body systems. The first page of the "Endurance Exercise Program" section features a table of pulse rates as percentage of max, from 60 percent up to 90 percent. Workouts are 20 minutes.

"You should strive to train about one day per week for at least ten minutes of your workout at 80 to 90 percent of maximum," the book advises. "This will help you improve at a rapid rate."

The progressive steps are set up so that you stay at each step until you can perform that workout regularly without going beyond 80 percent maximum heart rate, other than on that one day of 80 - 90 percent effort.

For the level at which I was coming into the program (i.e., at 19 mets), the first step (rated at 12.5 mets) has me doing 3.0 miles in 21:46, or at a 7:15 pace, certainly within my current capabilities. Step two is also reasonable; it calls for me to be putting out 13.1 working mets, running 3.0 miles in 20:54, or a 6:58 mile. Step three would be a little tougher, but still possible: 13.7 working mets, 3.5 miles, 23:16, 6:39 pace. I can see spending quite a few weeks at some of the levels.

The running program lists 24 steps, however. For the person coming in at one met, the computer extrapolates a sensible program. Coming in at 19 mets, step 12 has me doing 20.6 working mets, running five miles in 22:06, or a 4:25 pace. I'll be able to run with Alberto Salazar in future races; he set a world record of 22:04 for five miles in 1981.

Stage 13 has me going the same five miles in 21:08, a 4:14 pace. So long, Alberto, see you at the awards ceremony. Taking it to its ultimate silliness, the computer extrapolation has me, in stage 24, doing 36.1 working mets, running 8.0 miles in 20:15, for a 2:32 pace.

The running and bicycling program charts are backed by a training diary, which each client is encouraged to keep faithfully. "It's almost impossible to help them when they come in and complain that their program has broken down and they haven't kept a record of what they *did* do," George said.

Keeping a diary or journal is extremely important for a variety of reasons, including backtracking the cause of injuries or plotting the training that led up to a particularly good race.

Clearly, the fitness testing has revealed more about myself than I'd ever expected and the computer had made it possible in only a few hours. The road map to improving my body and my fitness was also drawn out by the computer. What I did after the testing, what roads I decided to take, was now entirely up to me. The computer had evaluated me.

But thoughts about all those tests kept nagging me inside. I was disappointed with the results of the immersion testing for body fat, true, but I was bothered by something else. I tried to pinpoint what was troubling me as I tied my laces for my daily run.

During the run it came to me. I was running relatively smoothly; my leg was twinging a bit, but as it warmed up the pain became less bothersome. I knew that I was in better shape than most people my age. But, at an almost subconscious level I was uneasy, restless.

As a kid I'd spent many a nickel in front of a pinball machine, intent on racking up enough points to get free games. After a few hundred nickels and developing a sensitive touch in the hands and wrists, I was racking up games almost at will. Once I had mastered the machine, the store owner would call the pinball company to have it carted away, to be replaced by a new machine with a more sensitive "tilt" mechanism. In a few days, however, I'd have that one licked, too.

I sensed a similar challenge from the treadmill at the S.M.A.R.T. Clinic. I'd got on it knowing that I was not in the best shape of my life, that I was injured, and remembered the words, "Don't try to beat the machine—it can't be done." Now I had the urge to get back into good shape, to "practice" by throwing in some good hills, to up the mileage, to become fit to go up against the treadmill again. All the apparatus they hung from the body was a nuisance—no boubt about it—but it wouldn't be as much of a diversion the next time.

I ran on, turning the idea over and over. And then I involuntarily laughed at myself; I realized that it wasn't the treadmill machine I wanted to overcome. I was merely using the treadmill to measure how well my own body could adapt to more training, more workouts, more careful development. I realized that I wanted to find out if I could move into stage seven, if I could elevate my VO_2 max by even a few points and if I could push the limits of my heart rate.

I knew I was fit. But fitness, like everything else, was only relative. How much more fit could I become? That, it seemed, was the on-going challenge. The treadmill was only a measuring device.

Ultimate fitness still lay beyond the far horizon. But my steps were leading me in that direction, even if in a roundabout way, with unscheduled stop-offs and detours. At least I was moving.

2

Going Nowhere Fast, Slow, Or In-Between
by Richard Benyo

There was a time in my life when I became fascinated by gerbils. I'd like to say that it was when I was a youngster, but it wasn't; it was more like when I was 30 years old. My childhood is never-ending.

Gerbils are small buff-colored rodents with white underbellies. They are on the species scale between mice and hamsters. But they are unlike any mice. Originally imported from Europe as lab animals for experimentation, the little critters were so cute and well-behaved that some lab assistants began taking them home as pets, bringing God-only-knows-how-many laboratory germs to the outside world. The gerbils found the new environment much to their liking, and their owners began breeding them. Soon, the gerbil population in this country escalated and they began showing up in pet shops.

The gerbil is unique in more ways than cuteness. While the mouse is promiscuous, the gerbil is Puritan. It is a very faithful creature. Once the male gerbil picks his mate he never leaves her. A pair of gerbils will not welcome the company of others.

Another advantage of gerbils over mice and hamsters is that their urine is odorless. They enjoy being handled and played with and they'll seldom bite—again, unlike mice and hamsters. They're kind of like civilized squirrels without the bushy tail; they have long, thin tails, and strong hind legs, and they are desert inhabitants.

So what does this dissertation on gerbils have to do with fitness? Plenty.

At the same time that I became interested in having a few gerbils as pets (which is a misnomer, because you can't just have a few gerbils as pets; they breed too regularly), a pet supply company began marketing the Habi-Trail. The Habi-Trail is an integrated system of plastic cages and connecting tubes that you can buy individually, or as a set, and connect so that they form a sort of city. You can put a chemically-treated handful of woodchips in the bottom of each one; there is a slot for a water bottle so the critters can drink without spilling; there are tubes everywhere through which the critters travel from one apartment to the next; there are turrets and towers and sleeping chambers and play cubes.

I bought the starter set and two gerbils, and later a sleeping chamber and a play cube. Then I bought another starter set. I was becoming a Habi-Trail junkie, spending a large percentage of my paycheck on plastic tubes, water bottles, wood chips and more and more living units. What started as a small cage was turning into a city; it spread all over my bedroom and ultimately headed out into the living room by a series of tubes that ran down the sides of my bureaus and across the floor under the bed. There were little grooves inside the tubes, so the gerbils could use them to walk uphill. Within a month, my two gerbils had the largest living quarters in Alexandria, Virginia. They had about a mile of connecting tubes and a dozen individual homes. I think that it had become too much for them, however. Going from a cramped cage at a pet store to a vast estate can disrupt the relationship of the most stable couple. The gerbils reacted in a very curious, but certainly a positive, stress-relieving way.

I forgot to mention one characteristic of gerbils that is common to most rodents: they are nocturnal creatures. What that means is that they are lethargic and sleepy during the day, but wide-eyed and active at night.

In the largest of the living cubes there was a plastic wheel. Every night, the two of them would head for that big cube, hop aboard the wheel that hung against the side of that clear plastic cube, and run their tails off. When one got off to get a drink of water, the other one would hop right on and take off. Frequently, both of them would be on it at the same time, one chasing the other in perfect formation. The first night with them in my bedroom was pretty disconcerting because I could hear their little clawed feet running like wild on the wheel. The second night it didn't bother me and I could sleep. But eventually, from using it about eight hours each night, the constant vibration wore out the clear plastic wall that supported the wheel. The treadmill began to wobble, but that didn't bother the gerbils. They merely adjusted to the wobbling and kept up their incredible long-distance running.

The wobble—and the noise—grew worse. I thought the police would come knocking at my door any night now, demanding that I stop the gerbils because of complaints from the entire apartment complex. I contemplated moving out of my apartment so that the gerbils could take it over and breed.

Actually, nothing like that happened. The people who made the Habi-Trail system conveniently sold replacement wheels. I bought a replacement unit and got some good sleep for several nights, until they wore that one down.

I began to wonder, with all the unique, interesting and catchy phrases in the English language, why no one had ever come up with this thought: as happy as a gerbil on a wheel.

I have never seen an animal as happy as a gerbil when he (or she) is pumping like crazy on a wheel. Gerbils love exercise, and although I never had their VO_2 max or resting heart rate checked, I'm sure that they were incredibly fit. They ate sunflower seeds and corn, took long naps during the day, drank a lot of water, but never really got fat. They worked it all off during the night.

Before I met the pair of gerbils, I had had some very negative feelings about treadmills and similar machines. Treadmills were places for going nowhere fast. They seemed to accomplish nothing. But, my thirtieth year was a revealing one, between learning conditioning from gerbils, and going through a very severe winter in the process of trying to lose weight and get in shape. Seeing how the gerbils enjoyed their time on the wheel and knowing that a local health club had two treadmills, I bundled myself up to face the cold and drove to Falls Church, Virginia, to meet my first treadmill.

THE BEAST IN ITS LAIR

As a kid, I was always torn between the outdoors and the indoors. I did not especially care for the "official" outdoors as espoused in *Outdoor Life*, where Woolrich-clad rabbit and grouse hunters went tramping around the woods looking for something to massacre, while expounding on their conservation efforts. But

I've always liked the woods. As a kid I used to roam through the woods, nosing around like a young raccoon, getting into occasional trouble with a bees' nest, an anthill, or a skunk that my friends and I thought we could capture and domesticate. (Liberal doses of tomato juice will get skunk stink off a kid that's been too curious.)

The outdoors was a place for me to explore or to look down on life from. I would run through the woods for a few hours, huffing and puffing like a pup, make it to the top of a mountain, and then sit back and look down on my home town, picking out my grandparents' house, friends, and occasionally my mom in the back yard hanging up clothes to dry.

A kid going outdoors is usually on a mission of some sort, real or imagined, and is therefore getting exercise. That's the big thrust these days with adults taking up strenuous outdoor exercises: they're getting back some of that unbridled freedom of movement.

Dr. George Sheehan, quoted in the last chapter, claims that children experience peak experiences every day, until they reach 13 years old, which is when they become freshmen in high school. Adults getting back into sports are becoming addicted to it, Sheehan feels, because they are once again having peak experiences, and they're liking it.

The outdoors has always had a sense of adventure about it. You never are certain that the weather isn't going to turn nasty on you. Often, the weather you are being exposed to is already pretty foul and you can set it up as an adventure from the first step. You are likely to take turns and trails you hadn't anticipated when you walk out the door, because there you have so many options. When you're a kid, the possibilities are even more massive because as a kid you don't necessarily need a path to follow: You're just as likely to push your way into a briar patch where no man has ever gone before.

I had an equal fascination with the indoors, however. Some might think that the indoors are very limiting, and in some ways they are—if you allow them to be. You obviously do not have the freedom to roam the wide-open spaces while you're indoors, but there are advantages: you have more control over your environment (so that it can be freezing outside and comfortable inside); you have some degree of privacy; you can more rapidly become familiar with your environment, and so on.

Being a kid who liked to read and who was fascinated by the

then-new diversion of TV, I enjoyed being indoors as much as I enjoyed being outdoors. I'd often closet myself in my room with a Hardy Boys book, until my father got suspicious of what was going on up there. When things got *too* quiet in the room I shared with my brother, this dialogue would ensue:
"What are you doing up there?"
"Nothing."
"What do you mean 'nothing'?"
"I'm not doing anything."
"People don't do 'nothing.' What are you doing?"
"I'm reading."
"Well, that's not 'nothing.' "
"I'm reading."
"Get dressed and get outside for a while. Get the stink blown off ya."

That was one of my father's favorite expressions. "Get the stink blown off ya." Like we were an armful of bedclothes that needed to be hung out to air.

So I'd dutifully (to avoid dire consequences; another favorite expression was, "I'll knock you into the middle of next week") stumble down the stairs, usually making too much noise ("How can a kid who weighs 95 pounds make so much noise?"), and I'd amble by my parents. I never got out the door without this, though:
"So what were you doin' up there?"
"Nothing. I wasn't doing nothing."
"Don't give me that."
"I was just readin'."
"Don't you have anything better to do?"
(I used to think of all kinds of wiseacre answers under my breath, but never owned the foolhardiness to utter them.) "I like to read," I'd say.

The storm door would close before I'd hear the final: "Go out and get the stink blown off ya."

So I went out and got the stink blown off me, thinking longingly where I'd left mean old Mr. Applegate about to do something to the Hardy Boys.

All of this is merely a preamble to being 30 years of age, trying to get back into shape, and facing a mighty cold day on the way to Falls Church and the local health club. I thought of my father as I walked to the car; the wind was whipping so hard that I was sure I was getting several days worth of stink blown off me.

When I first walked into the super-saturated air of the health club, I almost turned around to escape. It was intimidating. The uniformed attendants looked rather military, and the "regulars" strutting around with all their extra muscles hanging out, made me feel rather inferior. Unfortunately, I'd already signed the contract to use the place, so I wasn't going to let my money go down the sauna drain.

I was most interested in trying to get back into shape by running, and luckily the club had two treadmills pushed into one corner of the exercise room. They were on the same side of the room as the most formidable-looking, chrome-plated Universal machine, which meant that I'd be spending my time next to the bodybuilders. I was also made self-conscious because the entire room was one giant mirror; even the door to get to the locker rooms was covered with a mirror and it took me several visits to figure out which mirror the locker room was hiding behind.

At first I thought that the mirrors were there because they made the place look bigger than it really was. But I later learned that they provided a place for the musclemen to watch themselves flex their muscles.

I sheepishly walked out from behind the locker room mirror in my J.C. Penney gym shorts, my white T-shirt with a pocket on the left breast and my Adidas Countries. I felt like a moldy banana in a bowl of wax fruit. I made like I was re-tying my shoe, while I watched a 50-year-old, gray-haired fellow who had a potbelly and was using one of the treadmills. I didn't want to act stupid and get up on the other treadmill, turn it on, and have it drag me along the belt and underneath it—my constant fear when riding an escalator. It seemed easy enough. He was just jogging along. I stood up after tying my shoe and examined the treadmill, as though I were a repairman looking for something that wasn't working quite right.

Even though I was a complete novice at examining a real-life treadmill, I noticed right away that this treadmill was *used*. The belt was worn and beginning to fray. The few rudimentary instruments that were clamped to the front rail (which included a speed control and a timer) were dangerously close to falling off, and some of the rollers under the belt were apparently out of alignment, because one of them kept making a tortured squeak on each revolution.

I didn't want to interrupt the guy on the treadmill, because he seemed as though he needed the work he was getting in, but I couldn't help it. "Aren't these treadmills in pretty ratty shape?" I asked.

"At least they're running today," he gasped, continuing to look straight ahead into the mirror (as though expecting to see his pounds of fat melt before his eyes) while the treadmill made its obscene squeaking noises.

I put my fears aside and cautiously approached the other treadmill. It seemed innocuous enough. I got up on it and stood, feeling a little foolish. Examining the controls, I saw that there wasn't much of a mechanical challenge here, even for a guy who has trouble changing a light bulb. There was a speed control and a timer, and that was it. They were attached to the front rail and there were no side rails.

I straddled the thing, keeping my feet off the belt, and turned the speed control to low. It made some rumbling sounds before starting and moving at a pace equal to a very tired old man's shuffle. I stepped onto the belt, trying to get used to the feel of the rollers under the belt and having to balance myself off the ground. I found myself walking easily and turned the speed control up a bit, telling myself that no matter how bad this was going to feel, it was better than being outside in the howling wind.

I matched my pace with the speed of the belt, finally rolling from a walk into a run. I set it at what seemed a reasonable pace; the controls indicated it was 8 mph. I later learned it was actually about 5½ mph. I was just getting into the swing of the thing, keeping pace with the guy on the next treadmill, when I was nearly thrown off my feet. The belt had coughed, or sputtered, or something. It had momentarily lost power, as though there was a short somewhere. The lurch was just enough to throw me off. Being naturally clumsy, I spent the next five minutes trying to get back on and recover.

I had just brought myself back into equilibrium when I heard the guy next to me mutter, "That one always seems to sputter if you get it going too fast."

I shook my head in disbelief. "Ah, yeah," I said, "thanks for telling me that." I was now too pissed off at the machine to give it up, so I stayed on it, always conscious that it might try to throw me off at any moment. The rest of the run (which the timer indicated was 15 minutes long), was agony. My anticipation of the machine lurching again kept me tense. My legs tightened and became unyielding and knotted. During the entire 15 minutes on the machine, I only felt two more lurches but the anticipation of that next sputter was enough to ruin my first experience on the treadmill.

Carefully lowering myself off the machine, I realized that I had probably done myself more harm than good doing a workout on such a contrary device. The other one, I learned, had its own quirks, which included one roller two-thirds of the way back from the front that was coming loose, so that you had to run carefully, making sure you picked up your feet before they went over that roller. If you put any weight on it, it was like stepping into a pothole.

As I got more seriously into running, I would occasionally think back to those experiences on the treadmills at the health club, and find that the only thing I could compare them to was the night I tried to run 12 miles at 11:00 in a drizzle. The entire run was spent trying to avoid real and imagined cracks in the pavement. I came back from that run with legs as tense as tree trunks, and with an ingrained fear of falling on my face, breaking my nose and my glasses, and not being able to find my way home.

I had stopped at the office after the first day to see if the treadmills couldn't be repaired. "Oh, the repairman was just in yesterday. They're running perfectly," the smiling attendant told me. During my tenure at that club, I was never to see *him* on the damned things.

During the ensuing year the treadmills were out of commission at least half of the time. I was blaming the treadmills as well as the club at first, but once I got more familiar with the situation I laid complete blame on the club.

The health club's design emphasized the indoor pool, the coed dry sauna that overlooked the pool (and that was built of native rock and glass), the Universal weight equipment and the juice bar (which was lovely, but which was never open when I was there).

The treadmills were almost an afterthought or a concession to the boobs who were using the facility for a real workout. I can imagine their board of directors meeting conversation going something like this:

Director One: This agenda says that some of the newer members want a treadmill. That sounds reasonable.

Director Two: That's right. There's a running craze now and our customers don't want to train in the ice and slush outside, so they expect us to provide something for them to use inside, like a track or treadmills.

Director Three: Out of the question. We've used up our budget already on those pastel towels that we can rent for an extra ten cents per.

Director One: But won't there be a backlash from the new members if we don't do something? We depend on them telling their friends, who are potential members—the kind that quit a few weeks after paying their entry fees.

Director Two: It's this running craze. And there's a tradition that health clubs are supposed to have treadmills.

Director Three: Out of the question. We've used up our budget on black lights for the kiddies Saturday morning exercise classes so we can keep them out of the toilets; we don't want any more toilet paper rolls stuffed down the toilets, do we? We have to keep the brats occupied while their parents are here.

Director One: But we have to satisfy all those joggers with something. They don't seem too keen to use the weights. Our boys scare them away. We've got to offer more than a pool and chewing gum dispensers.

Director Two: Let them have their treadmill.

Director Three: Out of the question. We've used up our budget on new contract forms with smaller print. Let them run outside. I saw somebody outside running the other day. He didn't get hurt on the ice. If they wanna run, let them do it on their own time.

Director One: Let's dig into the slush fund and get them a low-ball treadmill. We can put it in the corner over by the locker room door.

Director Two: Don't forget, though, if we put one in the men's side, the women will scream for one, too.

Director Three: Out of the question. Women can't run. And I'm against dipping into the slush fund for anything. I don't want to have to fly coach class on our annual outing to Bermuda. Out of the question. Besides, I think it's against county ordinances to allow people to run inside a building. It's dangerous. And what if somebody falls off one of the things! We'll be sued and never get to Bermuda.

Director One: I have a friend who owes me a favor. I'll see if he can get us some used treadmills at a good price. Maybe we can get three or four for the price of one, as long as we go for quantity instead of quality—and don't ask to have them repaired when they break.

Director Three: Okay. No quality. None of those industrial-strength treadmills that elephants can run on and not destroy. There's no room for something like that here. Besides, they're too expensive. If you can get a few treadmills for the price of one used one, I'll just cut back on the extra luggage I take to Bermuda this time to make up the money. But this is it. After this, we leave the slush fund alone.

Director Two: This'll make the cardiorespiratory freaks very happy.

Director One: Now, let's get back to something serious. Let's hear about this proposal to have scented water in the showers and supported by a major advertising campaign...

That may not be an accurate representation of the way the treadmills came to be, but they very obviously were not given priority. Even I could see that. The two treadmills had to be plugged into one of those multiple outlets you plug into a baseboard outlet when you realize you've got too many appliances and not enough plug-ins. It was a fire marshal's delight. There were plugs and cords winding all over the floor in front of the treadmills. It was a good thing, too, the treadmill had front rails, because if you got going too fast, you could crash into the mirrors and land in a tangle of cords.

The models I was stuck with were by no means the industrial-strength style. I was sure they'd only been driven on Sundays by little old ladies. I decided to give them a chance anyway. *If* they were working during my visits.

They often weren't. I would come into the club, ready to play gerbil, only to find a barrier set up around them with a sign indicating that they were not operational. And when they were operational I'd usually find both of them in use, with a line of guys waiting for their turn. No amount of complaining would convince the owners to purchase newer, stronger treadmills or to add a few more.

Between the periodic breakdowns, the repairmen coming in to work on them, and the barriers strung up around that corner of the gym, it looked like heavy construction was underway. From the day I joined the club, until the day, a year later, when I transferred my membership, the same two machines were brutalized. By the time I left, the treadmills sounded like Sherman tanks on maneuvers.

There are many treadmills available today, some of them with as many options as a new automobile, and just as expensive. They come in all shapes and sizes, all price ranges, and from companies big and small. Some come already assembled, some come in hundreds of pieces that you can assemble. By assembling it yourself, you can save quite a bit of money—and you can learn firsthand how a treadmill works. Not that it's complicated.

I'll discuss the two basic types of treadmills, motorized and non-motorized, but first, I'll view the treadmill as an allegory on fitness.

FIT TO RUN

As I originally discussed about the treadmill, one of its negative connotations has always been the fact that you are working hard and going nowhere. People relate to ignorant animals that run on treadmills or inside exercise wheels, and they shake their heads in sympathy for them. People who do not like their jobs or who find them boring, refer to their work as "running on a treadmill." This saying infers that their job is a dead-end, and that they are going nowhere fast.

Not true. While you are going nowhere fast, you are accomplishing something. You are exercising. (I often envisioned heavy-duty treadmills, hooking them to a generator, and powering the club. It would reduce the electrical bill because there are plenty of guys anxious to get up on treadmills, ready to roll. Perhaps, with the impending power shortages, some modern-day Edison will hook up the proper apparatus to exercise machines throughout the nation and harness all that energy being expended.)

How many unfit gerbils have you seen? If they've stayed up all night using their exercise wheel, they're terribly fit, they sleep soundly and they have good appetites.

Fitness, I suppose, is like a treadmill.

You can expend quite a bit of energy achieving it, but in reality you are not accomplishing anything that is going to stop the world in its tracks. Your fitness however, is going to keep the world from stopping you in your tracks.

Ancient Greek long-distance runners used to cover a hundred miles or more in a day while delivering messages. They were certainly physically fit. But they were not doing what they were doing to be fit; they were doing it because it was a job that had to be done. Although you can gasp in astonishment at their accomplishments today, they were people who were held in rather low esteem in those days. They were merely messengers, probably equivalent to today's milkmen and paperboys. They did their work, they got their pay envelope at the end of the week, and they went out to see a double-feature Greek tragedy on the weekends—that was it. Imagine how fit they were. They didn't smoke because cigarettes hadn't been invented yet. They did drink wine, of course, but a half-bottle of wine a day has recently been shown to encourage the body's production of high-density lipoproteins, a factor that works against heart disease (see Chapter 1). I wonder how they treated strained Achilles tendons and sore muscles. No doubt they probably had some sort of poultices and medicines that took care of that. These runners were surely the fittest people of the Greeks.

He knew he'd put in a good day's work when it was over. His message-carrying was often life-saving. When the weekend came, he might take a busman's holiday by running about 60 miles to see his family in the town down the road.

To him, life didn't seem like a treadmill on which he was trapped. Working toward fitness puts you into a situation pretty similar to the Greek messenger's. No one is going to hang medals on you for the perspiration you generate in a day's workout; most people wouldn't care if you were fit. That's not at the top of their priority list. They're more concerned that you don't allow your dog to make a mess in their front lawn.

But the important thing is that you *would* be fit, and that fitness would have a profound effect on your life. Sure, the half-hour or hour a day that you would be devoting to your own personal fitness would seem like a waste of time to people not oriented to fitness. They might look at you and mutter under their breath: "Gee-whiz, what a profound waste of time. That person's really on a treadmill. What's all that effort and sweat going to accomplish?"

The scientific evidence mounts that what all that effort and sweat is going to accomplish is improved health, increase capacity to enjoy life, instill a purpose in life, and create a feeling of well-being. There is even evidence that it may prolong life, but whether or not it does is almost beside the point. Fitness for its own sake is often enough.

And fitness is certainly a repetitive process, a seeming treadmill (whether or not using a treadmill is part of the exercise program) that should never end.

But enough philosophizing. I'm going to look at the two basic types of treadmills and their many variations, pick one out for your use, and get into some fitness programs that you can begin with relative ease.

HUMAN POWER VS. ELECTRIC POWER

Treadmills are typically powered in one of two ways: by your running and moving the belt, or by an electric motor that moves the belt upon which you run.

The human-powered treadmills are generally less expensive than the electrical-powered treadmills. Both usually employ a series of rollers under the belt, and a bit of technique is called for to make them work effectively when you aren't using electricity. You must gain momentum to get them moving regularly, and master the process of keeping them going. On the motorized treadmill, the belt is moving and you merely run on top of the surface as it is going, adjusting it to whatever speed you wish. The motorized treadmill, of course, is quite a bit more expensive.

Before providing programs for the treadmill, I'll examine the pros and cons:

PRO	**CON**
Manual	
1. Economical to buy and maintain	1. Must learn new running technique
2. Easy to move and store	2. Must concentrate on technique
3. Easy to repair when broken	3. Can be thrown because of misstep
Motorized	
1. Easy to use	1. Costs range from $1200 to $6000+
2. Most are adjustable for angle of attack (i.e., hillwork)	2. Difficult to store conveniently
3. Adjustable speeds	3. Repairs often difficult

The question of what type of treadmill is best for you ranks right up there with questions such as: Should you go on your vacation to the mountains or the beach? Should you rent an apartment or buy a condo? Do you need the utility of a station wagon or do you want the fun of a sports car? And so on.

I'll take a look at each type, and perhaps you'll get a better idea of which (if either) would be best.

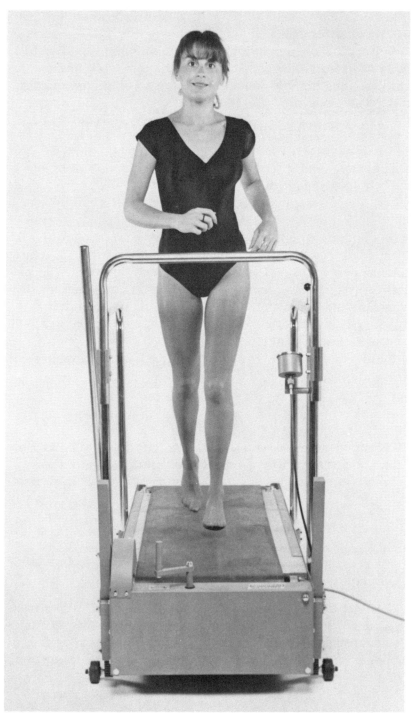
Pictured is the Trotter Treadmill, one of the most sturdy units on the market today.

PEOPLE POWER

There is something to be said for anything that runs without the aid of electricity or an internal-combustion engine. Bicycles, for instance, have a tremendous advantage when it comes to fuel savings; they are light, easily stored, easy to repair, and they provide the rider with a certain feeling of independence. They are also quite limited in their applications to the real world: It is difficult to bring home groceries for a family of four on a 10-speed bicycle, and even the most hardy of souls finds it difficult to treat a 100-mile bicycle trip to see friends as merely a lark.

There is something of the same feeling going when talking about the basic you-turn-it style treadmill.

If you are able to enjoy it with a genuine fervor, you will benefit greatly from it. A manual treadmill is relatively simple in construction and design, and if you are adept at balancing, you should have no trouble using it.

You just step up on the belt, grasp the support rails, and push off in a simulated walking pace, then roll into a running pace. You must make effective use of your toes on this type of machine, because the belt is designed for traction so that the toe of the shoe coming down on it, rolling onto the sole, in effect pulls the belt backwards. The act of running, as explained by some experts in human biomechanics, is a constant series of recoveries from near falls. You throw yourself forward and as you are about to fall, put out your foot to catch yourself. But instead of stopping to breathe a sigh of relief, you continue to throw yourself forward, catching yourself with first one leg, and then the other; put together, the series of falls becomes something that is easily controlled by yourself, and by practicing, you can do it blindfold. The use of the manual treadmill is very similar. It is like learning to have a rug pulled out from under you time after time until you are no longer surprised. Sound like fun? Maybe, if you're practicing pratfalls.

My findings have been that, much like roller skating, there are some people who find learning to run on the manual treadmill to be the height of simplicity, while others, like myself, find it almost impossible to master. I am not the most adept person at controlled body movements, and consequently, I have found it very difficult to use the manual treadmill.

Which may be safer in the long run. If I were able to get comfortable on it, my fear is that I would allow my mind to drift, as

I often do when I'm running, and on a manual treadmill, if you allow your mind to drift from running in the specific way that the treadmill requires, you are likely to lose your balance and fall. Luckily, the safety bars are high enough that they are easy to grasp if you slip.

I recommend that you go to a dealer and try out a manual treadmill before buying. Take along the clothes and shoes in which you do your workouts and give the unit a good test run before you even consider buying it. You may be one of those who has balance and agility and who finds it no trick to adapt to a manual treadmill.

Another shortcoming of the manual treadmill is its speed. It will go only as fast as you can run on it. In other words, you can't set it at a certain speed and practice your pace at that speed. In that sense, the manual treadmill approximates the real world—you run whatever pace you are telling your body to run. On the electric treadmill you can adapt your pace to a pre-set speed. Unfortunately, your pace-training is designed to teach your body pace, and not the other way around: you aren't trying to have pace come from within your muscles and breathing, because they do not yet know it well enough to dictate it effectively.

It is for these reasons that I'm going to suggest that you do not invest in a manual treadmill—unless you are quite capable of supreme feats of coordination and balance. And promise not to run too long on a manual treadmill to the point you become lulled into that comfortable sense of floating that running brings. You lose your balance very quickly on a manual unit in this state of mind.

POWER TO THE PEOPLE

After examining the features of a half-dozen motorized treadmills, I've settled on one that I feel is strong, serviceable, easy-to-use and economically priced.

We went out and examined treadmills from a little more than $1000 up to a "Star Wars"-like model in the $6000-range that literally did everything but resole your shoes while you were running on it. Ironically, the one we settled on was a mail-order model that was invented by a runner, Dick Trotter—a fitting name, indeed, for both a runner and a treadmill. (Trotter Treadmills, New Englander Industrial Park, P.O. Box 326, Holliston, MA 01746; 617/429-7676.)

Before getting started on putting together the program, I'll examine the unit.

The first impression you get of the Trotter Treadmill is its heavy-duty construction, a sort of industrial-strength treadmill. You'll recall my comments earlier on the treadmills that they had at the health club I joined. The Trotter is by no means beautiful. It has no fancy fiberglass aerodynamic panels to hide the stark corners, but it is totally functional and looks it: a Mack truck instead of a Triumph Spitfire.

The unit comes in three models: the C-22 kit, which you assemble according to more-than-adequate instructions, and costs $1195, the C-22 Standard, which comes assembled except for installing the rails and control bars, and which costs $1945, and the C-2100 Supreme, which features a motorized elevation control and other trick modifications, and which costs $2215. These prices are as of mid-1981 and subject to change. We got the C-22 Standard. It arrived by common carrier in a wooden crate shaped like a wedge of cheese with the tip snipped off. Assembly took about an hour.

The Trotters are available with up to six speeds, which range from a pedestrian 1 mph to 13 mph. Our unit was equipped with a 3.2-10;2 mph range. The unit features a 1.5-hp heavy-duty A/C motor, extra-strength side handrails, and a hand crank to elevate the angle of attack up to a 25 percent grade.

Peter Haines, the sales manager, put the unit's durability into perspective: "Since we deal direct with our customers, we had to build a unit that would survive the torture of the common carrier and perform flawlessly the first time it was turned on in Albuquerque as well as Anchorage."

Haines keyed on four favorable features of the treadmill:

1. The 1.5-hp motor operates at one constant speed regardless of the speed the running surface is traveling. This extends the motor's life.

2. The running surface is 1½-inch solid, laminated plywood. The top surface is birch, which has been treated with industrial Teflon. When used in conjunction with the custom-designed running belt, a most comfortable running surface with a low coefficient of friction is created.

3. Because of the availability of an inexpensive option of heavy-duty casters, the unit is very easy to move for cleaning or relocation.

4. Heavy-duty siderails provide the reassuring safety of protection, and an optional front handrail is also available.

The Trotter Treadmill doesn't offer any elaborate claims except that it is heavy-duty and has a long life, and if anything does go wrong with it, you can probably fit it with instructions and parts from the company.

This is not to say that the Trotter Treadmill is the only one worth buying. Some other units are quite sturdy and dependable. The Trotter struck us as interesting because of its direct-to-customer arrangement and its simplicity of operation.

This is how it works:

You mount the unit from behind, straddle the belt by standing on the sides, and survey your controls. There is a speedometer/odometer (that measures to the hundredths of a mile) on the left front rail, a start/stop knob coming through the left rail, and a speed control outside the right rail. In front of the unit there is a hand crank to elevate the running surface, but you can ignore that for the time being.

As you straddle the belt, make sure that the speed control is pushed all the way forward so that the belt will start up at the slowest possible speed (which in this unit is 3.2 mph). Next, simply pull up the start/stop knob on the left rail and watch the belt start moving. Now, step onto the belt (much as you would step onto an escalator) and walk briskly. Continue walking until you are completely comfortable with the speed. Now you can increase the speed to as much as 10.2 mph, which is just a hair under a 6:00 mile. Just pull back the speed control bar, which is located outside the right handrail.

As with any such equipment you purchase or use at a health club, practice with all of the functions until you become comfortable with them. Get to know all of the speeds. You don't want to be in a serious exercise session, throw a switch, and have the machine do something totally unexpected.

The Trotter is no problem to operate, and the surface is quite easy and smooth to run on; you can even use it barefooted.

Now that you've become used to the operation and various functions of the treadmill, I'll give some easy programs that build toward putting the treadmill to heavy use.

A RUN IS A RUN IS A RUN

A treadmill is as close as you're going to get to running indoors

Going Nowhere Fast, Slow, Or In-Between 71

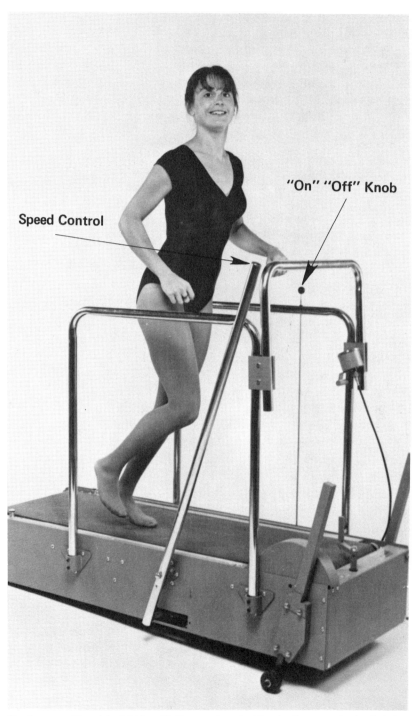

The bar near Rhonda's right hand is the speed control for the Trotter unit, the little ball near her left hand is the "Off" and "On" control.

and approximating running outdoors. Running on an indoor track is almost a sin against nature, and running around a gymnasium is likely to cause a whole raft of injuries.

I remember having to run around the inside of a gym as part of high school basketball practice. It still gives me the shivers to think of it. Since gymnasium floors are perfectly flat and have very defined corners, a kid is required to:

1. Take a pounding on hardwood floors.

2. Round tight corners on a flat surface, which puts tremendous strain on the ankles and knees.

Running on an indoor track is an improvement, but not much more satisfying, and not very accessible. Some gyms have running tracks around the upstairs balcony on the basketball court. They may even have tanked turns. They are often as much as 24 laps to the mile and you are usually dodging concrete pillars. Regular indoor competitive tracks (11 laps to the mile) are almost impossible to find, and if you do live near one, the people who maintain them won't let you run on them anyway. And besides, they're usually portable and they are set up only a few months of the year—during the indoor track season.

My most memorable "indoor track" was at the second health club I attended. It was a brand new club. Instead of the two overworked and underfed treadmills that were featured at the first club I joined, I guess they felt they'd save some electricity in the new place, so they put a "running track" around the outside of the weight-training room. It ran around the perimeter of the men's weight room. It was everything horrible that running around a basketball court can be, with sharp corners, hard floors, a narrow lane and people always opening the locker room doors on you unexpectedly. It was just about as unsafe as running on an interstate highway. I soon gave that up and began running on the roads. The management informed me that they had no intentions of getting a treadmill, because in the *total health facility* (which is what they called their new club), treadmills were passe.

When I first used the decrepit treadmills I became more patient. Just because the treadmill is a machine, and is safely tucked away in the intimate confines of your home, does not mean that it is capable of performing miracles for you. It does not do your running and any program of running, whether on the open road or on a treadmill, must be approached seriously. It goes without saying that there are more than enough running books on the market.

Going Nowhere Fast, Slow, Or In-Between 73

Between 1977 and 1980, there were probably more books written on running than on Hollywood celebrities. Some of the books are excellent, some are so-so and quite boring, and some are downright dangerous.

Most running programs can be easily adapted to the treadmill. You will have to read past all the inspirational passages about running with the wind (unless you set a fan on a chair in front of you as you run on the treadmill, which isn't such a bad idea, by the way).

I am assuming that, since you are into the *Advanced* aspect of the book's title, you are serious about getting on a treadmill and spending some time there. Since running on a treadmill and running outside are similar I will recommend some running books.

Jog, Run, Race by Joe Henderson, Anderson World, Inc.

Run Farther, Run Faster by Joe Henderson, Anderson World, Inc.

The Complete Book of Running by Jim Fixx, Random House.

The Complete Runner by the Editors of *Runner's World*, Anderson World, Inc.

Running for Everybody by the Editors of *Runner's World*, Anderson World, Inc.

Beginner's Running Guide by Hal Higdon, Anderson World, Inc. Inc.

Running the Lydiard Way by Arthur Lydiard with Garth Gilmour, Anderson World, Inc.

If you have been overweight and out of shape and are making a comeback, primarily through running, I'd like to suggest one of my books:

Return to Running by Richard Benyo, Anderson World, Inc. Good way to get in a plug, huh?

Anderson World, Inc. (see World Publications), is the sister company of *Runner's World* magazine and was publishing books on running long before the running boom hit.

But to repeat, approach running on the treadmill exactly as you would approach running outside: take it easy and work your way up to higher mileage gradually.

TREADMILL RUNNING 101

Start your program with a 10-minute workout that combines walking and running. The walking will accustom you to the treadmill's moving belt while warming your muscles at the same time.

Your first day should be easy:
> 3 minutes walking at the treadmill's slowest speed
> 5 minutes of running at 6 mph (i.e., 10:00 miles)
> 2 minutes walking at the treadmill's slowest speed

After you get off the treadmill, walk over to a wall and stand about two feet away while facing it. Keeping your body straight and your feet flat on the floor, lean toward the wall. Your hands will touch the wall, as though you were being frisked by the police. Keeping your body straight, lean into the wall and allow your nose to lean right up against it. Hold this pose for at least eight seconds. Feel the pull in your Achilles tendon. Return to a standing position. Now lift your right knee to your chest and then lower it; do the same with your left knee. Then lean into the wall again and hold it for a count of 10. Finally, walk around the room a few times.

The object of any exercise is to introduce some physical stress to the body, and then to work the body as much as you can to strengthen it to cope with stress. Jumping right into exercise and just as quickly stopping it adds strain on top of the stress. The parts of your body that have been exercised are frantically attempting to cope with things that are happening too fast for them. I often compare my own body to that of a dinosaur. The story goes that dinosaurs, because of their great size and tiny brains, could have their tails cut off and the message that they had lost them wouldn't get to their brains until the next day.

It is much the same with the human body. Before it is subjected to stress, it should be warmed to the task—which is why the walking phases on the treadmill are recommended.

The middle portion of the workout is when stressful exercise is best done and after that your body should be carefully returned to a resting condition. Once again, this is accomplished by walking.

Stretching after a workout is important for lengthening and loosening your muscles. Stressed muscles always contract. To see this first-hand make a fist and hold it for 60 seconds, very tightly clenched. When you open it, notice the reluctance of the muscles to respond smoothly. You can help your fingers return to normal by prying them apart and stretching them a bit beyond an open-palm position. The same is true of the exercising leg muscles—and of any other muscle in the body, including the heart, which should be given rest after it has worked hard.

While some stretching is good, I don't believe prolonged stretching is beneficial to your fitness. Yoga may make you extremely loose, but it does virtually nothing for strengthening your body or for producing aerobic benefits. Yoga should only be used to make your body work more effectively.

The wall stretch that follows your exercise on the treadmill is done to lengthen the hamstrings and the calves. In running, not all muscles are used. A stretching routine keeps the stronger leg muscles from completely overpowering the weaker leg muscles. The perfect prescription for exercise would be to work all the muscles in a series of exercises, but that is highly impractical right now.

TREADMILL RUNNING 102

The total of five minutes walking, five minutes running, and 45 seconds of stretching is about as basic as you can get, but it is a good starting point for the first week as you work to get familiar with the characteristics of your treadmill. You also have a chance to familiarize yourself with exercising on a machine and the feeling that a rug is constantly being pulled out from under your feet. It is best to be comfortable with the rug-puller before getting too ambitious with it. Don't worry if you take one or two days off the first week.

With something as convenient to use as a treadmill, it is my feeling that it should be worked into a regular schedule so that it can become a part of your daily routine. If you work Monday through Friday, work out on the treadmill during those days, taking Saturday and Sunday off. That way, just as your five consecutive days of work have become a constant in your life, so your exercising on those days can be fit into a little niche. Weekends are used as an escape from the regularity of the weekdays, and they should also be used to escape from the treadmill. If you are active on the weekend, do whatever it is you enjoy. Just stay off treadmills.

If your schedule is a little less rational, like co-author Rhonda's, you will still want to work at least five sessions with the treadmill into your week, placing them where they are convenient. Since Rhonda works some 24-hour shifts at a hospital and sometimes has two consecutive days off during the week, it would be impossible for her to follow a daily schedule. But a person who has a varying work schedule often knows a week ahead of time what the schedule will be, so it is possible also to plan workouts ahead.

For people like firefighters, who have almost totally unpredictable schedules, it might be best to get a group together and purchase a treadmill, install it in the firehouse and, between calls, do exercises.

When the emphasis is exercising on the treadmill five days a week, with two days off, you should tone down your intensity, as compared to doing your workouts every other day. With something that involves running, however, I've found that it is best to run as many days as are comfortable, because running in itself keeps you loose for the next day's run. Taking too many days off during the week will reduce your flexibility and compromise running's benefits.

It is not difficult to tone down on exercise programs using a daily schedule. Add a bit more walking and be more conservative about increasing distances or speed.

In the initial stages, while you are still getting used to the treadmill, and to your body's own adaption to it, it is best to keep the workouts the same every day. After several weeks you can begin varying your routine to simulate running outdoors.

Do the following daily workout beginning week two:

    3 minutes of walking at the treadmill's slowest speed
    8 minutes of running at 6 mph
    2 minutes of walking at the treadmill's slowest speed

Follow the exercising phase with more stretching of the hamstrings and calves, and also do some slow, very precise toe-touches. Following each of the stretches, take a slow, leisurely walk around the room to further loosen your legs. If you still feel bursting with energy, don't get back on the treadmill, because we want to have you easing your legs into that gradually. Instead, check chapters 3 and 5 and do a few (but not all) of the free exercises Rhonda outlines. As you get farther down the indoor road with your treadmill, you should supplement those workouts with some other types of exercise in order to develop your upper body.

TREADMILL RUNNING 103

By the fourth week of using the treadmill, you can begin a hard/easy format. Put in a hard effort one day, followed by an easy day that serves as a recovery time. Keep training daily to maintain consistency and to stay loose. Fit some activities into your weekend that allow you to use your increased fitness: bicycling, hiking, volleyball, skiing, just about any weekend activity will be enhanced by what you are doing for yourself during the week.

Here's the next several weeks' schedules, but I'll use shorthand from this point on. If I indicate "3mW" it will mean "3 minutes walking at treadmill's slowest speed." If I indicate "8mR6" it will mean "8 minutes running at 6 mph."

Your fourth week should work out something like this:

>Monday — 3mW/8mR6/2mW
>Tuesday — 3mW/10mR6/2mW
>Wednesday — 3mW/7mR6/2mW
>Thursday — 3mW/11mR6/2mW
>Friday — 3mW/8mR6/2mW

Your fifth week will have a little more variety by adding some speed:

>Monday — 3mW/8mR6/2mW
>Tuesday — 3mW/10R7/3mW
>Wednesday — 3mW/8mR7/2mW
>Thursday — 3mW/10mR7/3mW
>Friday — 3mW/8mR6/2mW

Your sixth and seventh weeks take another step up, but plateau to allow your body to catch up:

>Monday — 3mW/8mR7/3mW
>Tuesday — 3mW/11mR6/2mW
>Wednesday — 3mW/7mR6/2mW
>Thursday — 3mW/12mR7/3mW
>Friday — 3mW/6mR6/3mW

From this point on, you can put together your own schedule weeks in advance, according to how you feel and your recovery rate from workouts. Proceed at your own pace. No two people are physically equal so you should not feel obliged to lock yourself into someone else's program. Your program should gradually increase the workload, certainly, but don't overdo it.

The principles of training are simple: strain/back off/strain/back off/strain/take a day off. When you first try a longer running distance or a higher speed, do it only once during that week and do not add very much at any one time. On the other hard day that week, either keep it like it was the previous week, or even make it easier. You may also want to make the easy day after a new, harder day even easier than usual to give your body a chance to recover.

By week 10, your program may be something like this:
Monday — 3mW/9mR6/3mW
Tuesday — 3mW/13mR8/3mW
Wednesday — 3mW/8mR6/3mW
Thursday — 3mW/12mR7/3mW
Friday — 3mW/7mR7/3mW

Speed, distance and time are not the only variables when using a treadmill for exercise. There is one other, called "angle of attack." Which brings us to:

TREADMILL RUNNING 201

Running on a level surface is wonderful training for running on a level surface. If you are a track runner, level surfaces may be fine. But if you want to improve as fast as the next guy who is probably doing hillwork, you too are going to have to throw a few hills or steps into your training.

In running, the first part of your body apparatus that tires is the front of your upper leg. Lifting your legs begins to seem impossible; it's as though there is some invisible creature hanging onto them, pulling them toward the ground. As your upper legs tire, your speed drops. The higher you can lift your leg (within reason), the longer it will be airborne while your momentum carries you forward, which will account for a longer stride and mean more distance covered between footfalls, hence more speed. (There are, after all, only two ways to increase speed: take longer strides and keep your leg speed the same, or take the same size stride and increase your leg speed.)

The most effective method of increasing stride length and of maintaining knee lift is to do hillwork or run stairs. Running stairs can be incredibly dangerous, because when you go up, you are exerting a great deal of energy and using a tremendous amount of oxygen. By the time you make it to the top of the stadium steps, you are lightheaded and gasping, you probably can't see straight, and your balance is a bit off. When you turn around (i.e., make a 180-degree turn) and come back down the steps, your equilibrium is all but gone and what do you see before you when your eyes focus but what appears to be a cliff? Stairs can play havoc with your sense of balance and after a few repeats of them, your balance is going to be so poor that you won't even know it if you miss a step and fall off into eternity. My cross-country team used to run steps when I was in college, and even running small sets, one guy tripped and was injured.

In doing any type of hillwork, though, one of the negative factors built into it by nature and the laws of physics is this: whatever goes up must come down.

Coming down is usually much more destructive than the effort to run up. Coming down a hill (or a set of steps indoors) your legs take a pounding. Muscles in the legs you don't normally use are pressed into service and you must constantly strain to maintain control. The famed Dipsea race (run over a mountain) from Mill Valley to Stinson Beach, California, each June, is known for its horror stories of runners who spend three days after the race walking down steps backwards because their legs are shot from the pounding they received on the treacherous downhills. The legs can take such a beating coming downhill that you'll be unable to run for days following the effort. That's why when running downhill you should remember the virtues of patience. Run slowly, walk if you have to.

The treadmill has a tremendous advantage in this regard. Whether or not it is equipped with a device to raise and lower it, the treadmill can be set up to feature an increased "angle of attack." "Angle of attack" is not a term that is meant to intimidate you. It merely means that the treadmill surface is angled so that you are running up what amounts to a grade.

On a treadmill that features an adjustment (either electrically activated or using a manual crank), there is almost always an indicator that will tell you the percentage of grade. On treadmills that do not feature such an adjustment, all you need is a few strips of plywood, two sets of coasters or some old newspapers. Lift the front of the treadmill and slip in whatever thickness you need to get the desired lift.

The addition of an angle of attack to a treadmill training program should be done the same way you are doing everything else, gradually. Don't jump right into such a radical angle so that you need climbing rope to hold yourself on the treadmill. To begin with, raise the treadmill a degree or two. That may sound rather conservative, but after a few minutes of using the treadmill with even this shallow angle, you will begin to notice the difference—probably in your thighs.

You should also apply the hard/easy training concept to elevating the treadmill. Train at a few degrees one day, and place the treadmill on level ground the next. The slant will increase the pull

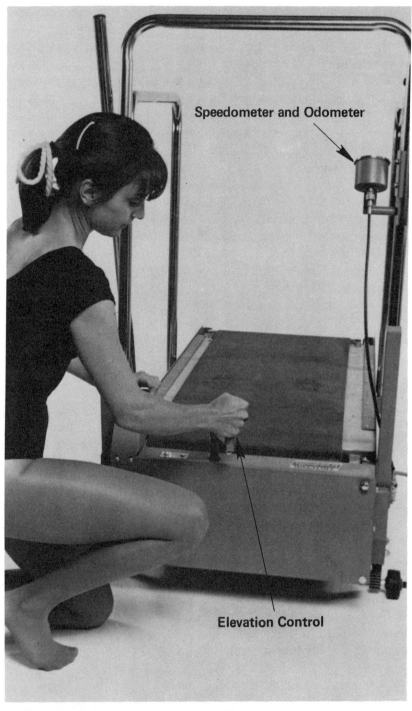

The Trotter has an easy-to-use handle for adjusting the angle of attack; their top-of-the-line model has an electric control so you can adjust the angle while running.

and strain on the Achilles tendon and calf. You should not want to apply too much strain at first.

Here's a program with a little lift that will pick up from week 10's schedule:

Monday — 3mW/9mR6/3mW

(use a level setting when there is no indication at the lead notation for a percentage of elevation)

Tuesday — 2%/3mW/13mR8/3mW
Wednesday — 3mW/8mR6/3mW
Thursday — 2%/3mW/12mR7/3mW
Friday — 3mW/7mR7/3mW

The 2 percent lift is by no means radical, so there is little concern in keeping the program identical to the 10th week except for the increase in elevation. Once you begin introducing more radical lifts, however, it will be advisable to cut back on the duration of the hard workouts until you become comfortable with the lift.

TREADMILL RUNNING 202

Here's a week 12 workout to illustrate the way you can work in more lift by trading off some length of workout:

Monday — 3mW/8mR6/3mW
Tuesday — 4%/3mW/10R8/3mW
Wednesday — 3mW/6mR6/3mW
Thursday — 4%/3mW/9mR7/3mW
Friday — 3mW/7mR7/3mW

Perhaps by the 15th week, you'll feel comfortable enough with moving back up to the lengths of workout you were using in the 10th week, even though you'll be at 4 percent lift on Tuesday and Thursday. Remember that all advances should be balanced by some additional easy days to allow your body to compensate for the increased stress load. For instance, when you do come back to the full 10th week workout with the 4 percent lift in the 15th week, you may want to have the Wednesday workout something like this:

Wednesday — 3mW/6mR5/3mW

The addition of easier days to help you successfully make advances in your hard days is not effort lost. You will be running a few minutes less for the week, but the week's energy output will be greater than it was when you were running your 10th week schedule on even ground.

TREADMILL RUNNING 203

From this point on, you should be able to sit down and come up with your own schedule a week or two in advance. Base your workouts on how you are adapting to the training. If you feel aches and suspicious twinges in the muscles, don't go rushing off into a new week with unusually high goals. There will come a time at the end of some week when you realize that you can't face another increase in your training. When that happens, you can do one of three things:

1. Keep the next week's training program the same as the week you've just finished in order to give your body a chance to reach a plateau. You may eventually feel comfortable at this level, in which case you can proceed to the next.

2. Drop your program back to that of the previous week. The drop back is merely an application of the hard/easy theory again, only this time on a week-to-week basis, instead of a day-to-day schedule. By dropping back at times you can actually make more long-term gains. This is an application of the battle strategy many great generals have used: retreat, regroup, and prepare to fight again.

3. Miss a day of training in the upcoming week. Perhaps you need a longer rest than just the weekend on this particular week to get you back on track. You may want to take Monday off. My preference would be to drop Wednesday. That way you will not have gone three days without working out. When I take three days in a row off, I find that on the next day back, my body is stiff and out of sorts.

Do not feel as though the schedules I've presented, or that the ones you come up with, are carved in stone. Changes can be made. Just do not begin to arbitrarily make deletions or changes when they are not really needed. It is too easy to fall back into the habit of inactivity.

TREADMILL RUNNING 204

Now comes the critical question in this program, and it is not something you should attempt to answer if you are merely reading this book through the first time and have not yet embarked on the program. Save this question until you're 15 weeks into the program:

"Just how fit is fit, and how far do I want to go with this program, anyway?"

Very good question. I'm glad you asked it. Only you can answer it. So much of your answer depends on your personality, how well you've adapted to what you've done so far, your goals and how much time you have to work out.

I've known people who have been the exemplary employees and worker for years, very responsible people, who took up a form of fitness (running, bicycling, etc.) and became obsessed with it, to the extent that they lost their jobs, their families, even—and this is subjective on my part—their sanity.

Competing in triathlons (for instance, a 2-mile rough-water swim, followed by a 120-mile bike ride, followed by a marathon run) does not make you fit. You become fit the first 15 minutes or so of your daily training. Everything beyond that is excess, self-gratification and straining for a goal. To some extent, it is a groping for the ideals of the wide-world-of-sport.

I'm not going to criticize such people. I'd be a hypocrite if I did. I've done my share of seemingly silly things that I still feel deeply satisfied about from having lived to describe them. Fifty-mile mountain races where you have to climb on hands-and-knees. Twenty-four-hour track runs.

The problem with such grueling occasions is that they can intimidate you from wanting to be fit.

Every time I do something like that, or hear someone else talking about an event that was outrageous or that required as much will power as muscle power to drive the person through it, I smile inwardly at the tenacity of human beings and at their profound silliness. Then I file it away in my memory somewhere and pretty much ignore it unless called upon to regurgitate it, as when a friend says, "Hey, do you remember the time that so-and-so ran a Triple Dipsea?"

If you're going to be happy and contented becoming fit, you've got to adopt the same philosophy. If all you want from your ambitious indoor exercising program is to become fit, so be it. Fit your workouts into your daily schedule, stick to them, smile while you're doing them, and enjoy the results. There is no need for you to run marathons or climb high mountains to become fit; and there is no reason for you to be intimidated by those who do things like that.

"Treadmill Running 204," then, concerns itself merely with: How far is far enough for me?

As we've already mentioned, about 15 minutes of steady aerobic workout about four days a week is going to provide you with all the health benefits you can expect from an exercise program. In just 15 minutes you're not going to have much time to move from one piece of apparatus to another or from one exercise sequence to the next. Fifteen minutes goes fairly fast if you are working at a steady pace. Ideally, with the warmup and cooldown tacked on the ends, you can be fit for a mere 20 minutes four days a week. What could be simpler? Some mornings it probably takes you that long to find your shoes.

If everyone in the United States donated 20 minutes a day to his own health and fitness and gave up smoking, heart disease could probably be cut down to about 10 percent of what it is currently.

For some people, however, mere fitness—once they get into exercising—isn't nearly enough.

It is ironic to see some people who are highly competitive in their business and personal lives get into exercise and merely use it as an outlet for their pent-up frustrations and stresses. But, on the other hand, some people with backgrounds that indicate they are sissies and totally non-competitive get into exercise programs and their personalities reveal a hidden face. They begin doing more and more exercise until they can literally scale tall buildings without breaking a sweat and they can regularly astound their friends and family with feats of wonder.

My attitude is this: more power to both of them!

An exercise program is totally adaptable to what *you* want from it.

If you want basic fitness, fine, it's there.

If you want to conquer worlds, fine, too—you're capable of doing it.

The following can be skipped by those who wish to work for basic fitness and maintain it.

TREADMILL RUNNING 301

Treadmill running is as close to outdoor running as you're going to get indoors. And, if you've got the dollars to pay for the electricity to keep it running for extended periods of time, you can most certainly do long-distance workouts on it. Some years ago a runner, at the opening of a new running shoe store, ran on a treadmill outside the store on the sidewalk until he'd covered a marathon. He ran it in something like 2:35—it was the world treadmill marathon record—and could have gone faster except that the treadmill didn't go any faster. I don't know what his electricity bill was. Actually, the average treadmill doesn't cost much in terms of electricity.

If it's storming and snarling outside, why turn your training into a pain in the ass when you can go out to the garage or down to the basement, flip on the treadmill and get in your workout? If you have stereo headphones, you can slip them on and run along to the beat. There is no reason you can't do a 20-mile workout in your basement on a foul Saturday morning. If you have the washer and dryer there, you can even do a load or two of wash while trotting on the treadmill. Your running shoes will last much longer, too, because the uppers won't begin falling apart from having been run through puddles and mudholes.

Any super-ambitious running program done on a treadmill should be approached just as it would be if you were doing a regular running program. Everything must be done in a logical progression.

There is no reason, though, that after three or four months of working out faithfully on the treadmill, you can't be doing a week like this:

        Monday – 5%/3mW/15mR7/3mW
        Tuesday – 10%/3mW/50mR7/3mW
        Wednesday – 5%/3mW/20mR6/3mW
        Thursday – 10%/3mW/75mR7/3mW
        Friday – 5%/3mW/15mR7/3mW

From there, it is a mere stretch of the imagination until you get up to:

        Monday – 8%/3mW/25mR7/3mW
        Tuesday – 15%/3mW/90mR8/3mW
        Wednesday – 8%/3mW/30mR7/3mW
        Thursday – 17%/3mW/120mR9/3mW
        Friday – 9%/3mW/30mR8/3mW

Beyond that, the unique language we're using here to indicate the workouts can be twisted and molded to fit anything you're ready for. You can even tell jokes in the workout language. How about this one?

        -6%/3mW/1500mR12/3mW

That's a pretty funny one, isn't it? That's accomplished by coming home drunk one night, putting a 6 percent wedge in the rear of the treadmill instead of the front and then keeping your time by the clock on the church tower down the street instead of by using a stopwatch. After you're done with it, you're guaranteed a classic case of shinsplints and you'll be out of traction in about two years.

Seriously, though, the treadmill offers a full slate of workouts. Your imagination, your common sense and your current state of fitness are your only boundaries. Climb aboard, turn it on, and get fit in the comfort and security of your own home.

3

Keeping All Systems Flexible
by Rhonda Provost

As I mentioned in my introduction, there are three basic components to fitness: strength, endurance and flexibility.

The promotion of strength comes primarily from trying to move weight, whether it be barbells or a pile of yesterday's newspapers. Endurance is derived from aerobic forms of exercise. (Chapter 6 deals with strength, and chapters 2 and 4 with endurance.)

I will discuss flexibility in this chapter and Chapter 5—that ability to bend or flex the body without injuring it. The idea is to learn to bend and flex more easily to gain a greater range of motion.

In doing flexibility exercises, you coax your body into assuming near-maximum positions in order to extend your limits. In the process of doing these exercises, because you are moving yourself against yourself, lifting your own weight so to speak, you will also gain some strength. That's because you are moving your own weight in a controlled repetition. Additionally, in exercise routines that continue beyond 10 minutes, you gain some endurance because you are gradually fatiguing yourself. So, even in exercises that concentrate on flexibility, we do venture, at least casually, into the other two areas of fitness.

Your body is a complex homeostatic mechanism. This means that everything that joins to form the body mechanism, down to the cellular level, strives to reach a state of equilibrium. Our bodies must maintain this state of equilibrium in order to assure survival. Disrupt the quilibrium over a certain timespan and the body systems begin to break down.

This need for equilibrium extends beyond the chemical level to the skeletal and muscle systems. The skeletal and muscle systems work together to safely house and protect all of your vulnerable internal body organs, and to give you mobility. Mobility, in fact, may be the most important single contribution of these two systems to the rest of the organism.

Movement, although centered on the skeletal and muscle systems, involves virtually every other system within the body. Some body movements are completely internal and contribute to your ability to both move and to live. These include the heart muscle, which pumps blood throughout the body to provide tissue with nutrients, oxygen and the intestines, which draw nutrients from the food we eat and expel that which cannot be used or that has already been used and must now be ejected as waste.

Our ability to move has been essential to man's survival. In prehistoric times, cavemen joined to get a fellow tribesman out of the path of a charging wooly mammoth. Today, getting up to move out of the direct path of a chill so that you do not catch pneumonia helps you to survive, as does the ability to quickly remove your body from the path of an onrushing bus. Your harmony with your environment, in fact, hinges on your ability to move away from undesirable situations and toward favorable ones.

Having spent years working with debilitated, bedridden or paralyzed individuals, the importance of muscle function has been brought home forcibly to me. We so often take even the most elemental body movements for granted, and too few of us work on refining and strengthening those movements. But imagine what life would be like without that great gift of movement!

Before getting into the flexibility exercises, I'll take a moment to consider the skeletal and muscular systems.

You've all seen skeletons jumping at people from dark closets, or cavorting in graveyards on Halloween night, or standing at attention in laboratories. The apparition of a skeleton holding itself together is either fanciful or contrived. A skeleton on its own is merely a bag of bones that would fall to the ground. Bones stick together and stay upright because something helps them.

Although it provides the framework upon which the rest of the body is built, the skeleton is able to support itself only through the complicated and marvelous attachment of muscles, tendons and ligaments, all of which provide a kind of flexible bonding. This wonderful structure of connecting materials, supporting buttresses, joints and levers causes the most talented structural engineer to shake his head in amazement. There is nothing simple about the human body, yet there is nothing complex—at least when dealing with the skeleton.

The muscles attached to the bones also cause the skeleton to move. The ligaments provide a flexible connection at the points where the bones meet (joint) and need to move.

Muscle tissue itself is characterized by contractility, extensibility, and elasticity. Contractility enables a muscle fiber to shorten and thicken. Extensibility enables the muscle fiber to stretch. And elasticity enables the muscle fiber to resume its original length, thickness and shape after the force stretching it is removed.

These three characteristics working in unison allow muscles a wide range of functions, and protect the muscles from rupturing with use. Being parts of a great machine, the muscles must be used in order to maintain—or improve—their function. If they are not used, they atrophy, and then when they are called upon to function, they perform poorly or not at all. But by using our muscles regularly, we will guarantee their continued smooth functioning. This fact becomes much more important the older we get, because aging causes joints and muscles to decrease in efficiency. The aging process is primarily chemical, and we have no magic pill to stop it. But by exercising regularly you can retard the aging process.

Besides making you mobile, the muscles are responsible for your ability to maintain posture and they produce most of your body heat.

Posture is the position of the parts of your body in relation to each other, regardless of your current position. Perfect posture would be the most relaxed and efficient alignment of all body parts possible in any given situation.

Muscles are responsible for posture—whether it be good or bad. They are primarily capable of just one function: contraction. A muscle contracts when your mind tells it to do so; the stimulation to contract comes from messages sent along the nerves, and is performed through the use of certain chemical substances that are present in the body. Because muscles can only contract (i.e., move in only one direction), they are arranged in groups of opposing pairs. If they weren't arranged in groups, you would be able to contract each muscle in your body only once in your lifetime, because there would be no opposite muscle to contract and pull the stretched muscle back to its original position. Your ability to maintain a posture, then, is the result of all your muscles (no matter which direction they are capable of contracting) receiving simultaneous messages from the brain (via the nerves) and circulating chemicals, resulting in a delicate balance of partially contracted muscles all over the body that allow you to stand, sit, or assume any of a thousand positions.

Good posture is an alignment of body parts that enables them to function at maximum efficiency. Good posture is also a state of balance that places the least amount of strain on muscles, ligaments, tendons and bones. Consequently, good posture should require the least expenditure of energy in order to maintain it.

Bad posture, on the other hand, places undue strain on any of a variety of organs, and robs the body of its potential efficiency. This improper alignment, if persistent, can lead to abnormal functioning of the various organs of your body, with resultant discomfort or poor general health. Bad posture can adversely affect your breathing, circulation and digestion. If, for example, you stand with your shoulders slouched forward, you are pressing down on the lung cavity, preventing the lungs from expanding to capacity, and therefore restricting their proper function. Long-term bad posture, especially if begun in childhood, can cause malformation of important body parts, and can subsequently cause injury to the nerves, muscles and vital organs.

It was mentioned earlier that muscles are the major producers of body heat. Each muscle, in order to contract, requires expending energy. When you send a message through your nerves and body chemicals for your fingers to strike typewriter keys, as mine are doing now, they perform that function by your body releasing energy (nutrients being converted to energy through the presence of oxygen). Energy released causes heat. Your muscles, even when at rest, provide much of the heat that keeps your body temperature consistent with your needs. (You can see the relation between muscle contraction and heat when you are standing in the cold and you begin to stamp your feet or flap your arms around yourself. Shivering is also a way for your body to generate heat.

Your body, the marvelous machine that it is, has a companion system (the pores) that will attempt to equalize your body temperature when you begin using your muscles vigorously; by creating perspiration, your skin is working much like an automobile's radiator, throwing off heat to the surrounding atmosphere. This system, like the muscle system, can be made more effective if it is used regularly.

The following exercises can be performed alone and without elaborate equipment. They can work both the muscle and cooling (perspiration) systems of the body. Because of their simplicity, they provide a ready means for improving posture, body control, and general body health. The three muscle groups responsible for good posture are the abdominals, back and leg muscles, so the exercises concentrate on those groups.

Some of these exercises will seem simple or repetitious, but they are included as a warmup before moving into the more ambitious portion of the routines. Even though this book is about advanced exercise, you don't ignore the need for warming up properly. You should notice that as you gain experience and familiarity with these exercises they will become easier and your movements will be smoother. This regimen takes about 30 minutes. At first, you may not be able to do all the exercises in the prescribed time. If you can't, that's just fine. Don't push yourself. As you become more comfortable doing them, they will take less and less time. Work at a brisk pace, and don't rest much between exercises. Concentrate on pacing yourself so that the exercises are comfortable. If some of them are too difficult the first time, go through the motions gently, and move on to the next one. Try the more difficult exercises again on your next session; eventually you'll master them. Technique is more important than speed. Save the challenge of the 30-minute goal for the point when you are doing all of the exercises comfortably.

I. Bend'n'Stretch—Standing, with legs apart about 18 inches, hold your arms straight out to your sides. While keeping both arms and legs straight, turn left and bend at the waist, touching your right hand to your left foot. In a smooth motion, resume the standing position, and from there, continue through to touch your left hand to your right foot. Repeat 20 times.

Then, in the same fashion, proceed to touch your right elbow to your left knee, return to standing position, and then continue through to touch your left elbow to your right knee. Repeat 20 times.

Complete the entire series twice.

II. Squat'n'Stretch—Begin by standing straight, with your legs and feet together. Now, squat down to the floor, bending at the knees. Place your hands flat on the floor on either side of your

Bend 'n' Stretch

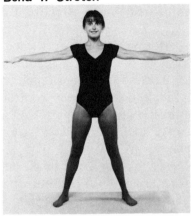
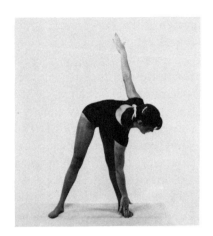
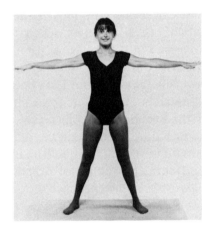

Begin by putting arms out to sides, then touch right fingers to left foot (above), coming back into the standing position (left), and then touch left fingers to right foot, returning to standing position. Then (below) put hands to back of head and prepare for next segment of sequence, illustrated on next page.

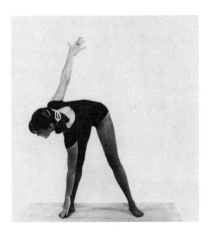
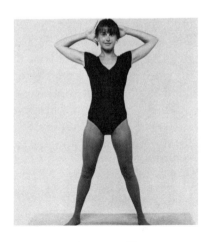

cont'd next page

Bend 'n' Stretch (cont'd)

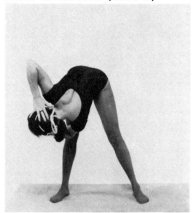
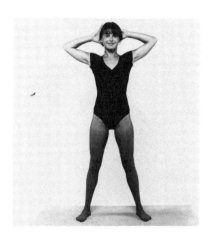
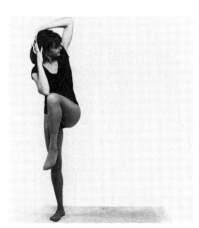
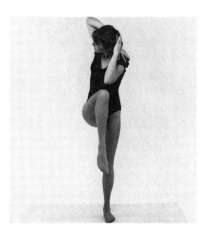

Alternately touch elbows to opposite knees, returning to standing position each time. Then, alternate bringing knees up to elbows.

feet. Bounce gently twice; then, while keeping your hands on the floor, attempt to straighten your legs as though you were going to stand. Hold for a count of three, being careful to bend from the hips, and not from the back. Return to the squat. Repeat 20 times.

When you are done, grasp your ankles and attempt to rise, straightening your legs; maintaining your position, try to touch your nose to your knees. Hold to the count of 10. Return to your standing position.

III. Sit'n'Stretch—Sit on the floor, with your legs spread far apart, forming a "V." Hold your arms out straight in front of you, keeping your back straight and your stomach in. Bend at the waist,

Squat 'n' Stretch

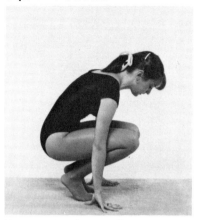 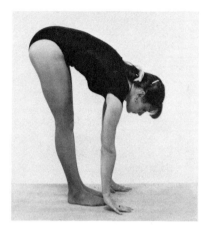

Keep your hands on the floor and stand up, attempting to straighten your legs. You may not be able to get the legs straight at first; if not, be patient: it'll come eventually.

and bounce gently four times to the center, going down as far as you comfortably can. Come back up, and repeat this stretch four times toward your right foot, then switch to your left foot and do four times.

Now, sitting straight up, put your arms out to your sides. Turning at the waist, try to touch your right hand to your left toes, while holding your left hand outstretched behind you for balance. Return to the upright position. Now, attempt to touch your left hand to your right foot, again bending at the waist, your right arm outstretched behind you. Return to the upright position. Repeat eight times.

Repeat the entire sequence four times.

Sit 'n' Stretch

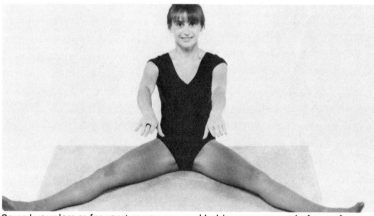

Spread your legs as far apart as you can, and hold your arms out in front of you.

cont'd next page

Sit 'n' Stretch (cont'd)

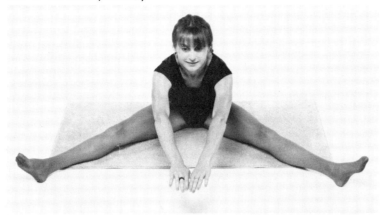

Reach for the floor as far in front of you as you can possibly stretch.

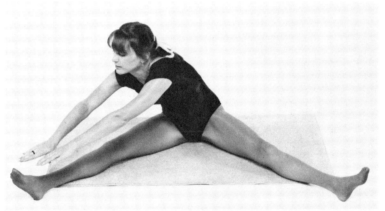

Then reach your arms out to your right toes, keeping the legs straight.

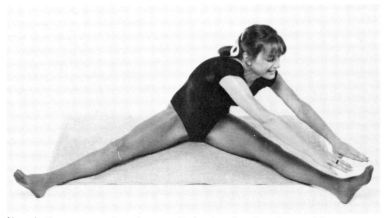

Now do the same stretch to the opposite leg, keeping those legs straight.

cont'd next page

Sit 'n' Stretch (cont'd)

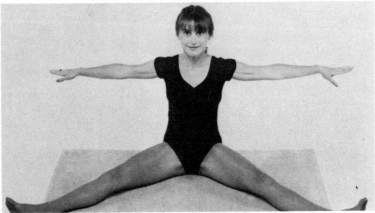

Now put your arms out to your sides, continuing to keep your legs straight.

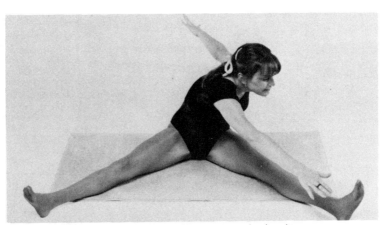

Then alternately reach for your toes with your opposing hand.

IV. Equilibrate—Equilibrium is the balance between opposing forces. This exercise involves a certain balance between opposing muscle groups. Sit on the floor with your back straight. Draw the sole of your left foot as close as possible to your crotch. Stabilize it there by holding it with your left hand. Now, grasp the sole of your right foot and extend your right leg up and out to the right. Repeat this 20 times. When finished, switch and draw the sole of the right foot in to the crotch. Hold it there with your right hand. Now, grasp the sole of your left foot and extend it up and out to the left side. Repeat this 20 times. Now draw both feet in to your crotch and grasp the soles of both feet simultaneously. Extend both feet up and out 10 times. Now do the entire sequence again.

Keeping All Systems Flexible 97

Equilibrate

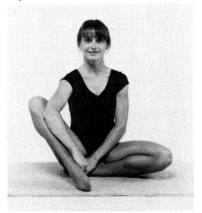
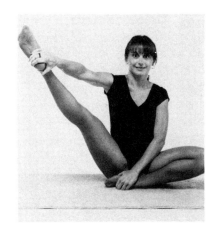
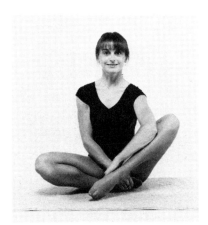
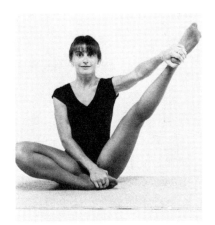
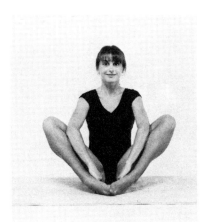
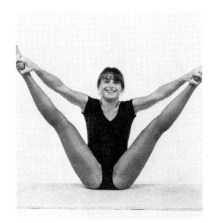

The secret with this one is to relax and don't try to stretch yourself beyond your body's inherent flexibility on the first try.

V. Thrust'n'Stretch—Sit on the floor, with your legs spread far apart, forming a "V." With your back straight, place your hands on your hips. Make a circle with your right hand, bringing it behind your back, and up over your head as though you were a baseball pitcher, touching your right hand to your left foot, attempting to touch your nose to your left knee at the same time. Bend at the waist. Then, bring your right arm back up in the reversed pitcher's throw, and allow your hands to land behind you, palms on the floor. You've now got four contact points with the floor: your feet and your hands. Concentrate on keeping the soles of your feet flat on the floor, and your palms flat behind you on the floor, and lift your body off the floor, thrusting your

Thrust 'n' Stretch

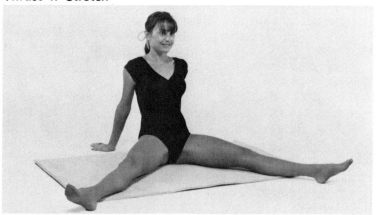

Keeping the legs straight is important in these exercises.

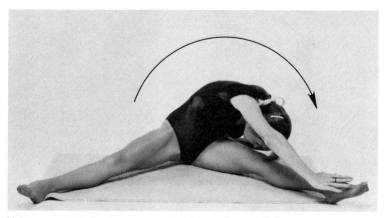

Make an exagerated swing over your head toward your left foot.

cont'd next page

Thrust 'n' Stretch (cont')

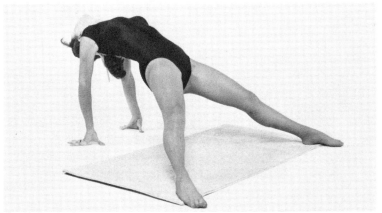

Having come back with your arms behind you, lift yourself off the floor.

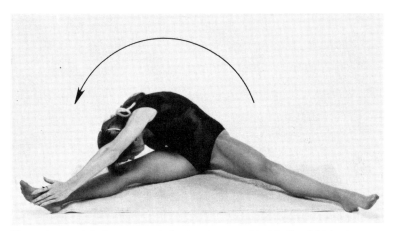

Then return and do the exaggerated swing over your head to the right foot.

pelvis toward the ceiling, bending your head back as far as possible. Lower your pelvis back to the floor and resume your original position. Then use your left hand, this time to bring it over your head, and touch it to your right foot.

Repeat the entire sequence 15 times.

VI. Variations on a Theme—Assume a sitting position on the floor, leaning back on your elbows and forearms. Maintain this position throughout this exercise. All the exercises will center on the legs and abdomen; your hands and arms are used merely to widen your base of support. Stretch your legs out in front of you, keeping them straight and together. All of the exercises that follow should ultimately be done with your legs straight, and your heels about four inches off the floor. If this is too difficult at the beginning, though, you can give them a brief rest on the floor when between exercises.

A. Hold your legs straight and four inches off the floor. Now, spread your legs apart as far as they will go, for a count of one, and bring them back together in front of you on count of two. Repeat eight times.

B. Hold your legs straight and four inches off the floor in front of you. Now, draw them up to your chest. Then raise them (still keeping them together) straight above your head, and then lower them *slowly* to the starting position. Repeat eight times.

C. Hold your legs straight and four inches off the floor. Now

Variations on a Theme

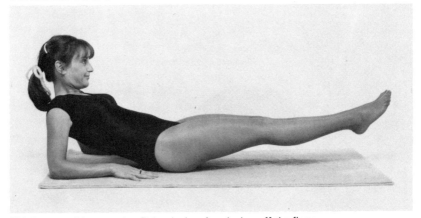

This is a very tiring exercise. Raise the legs four inches off the floor.

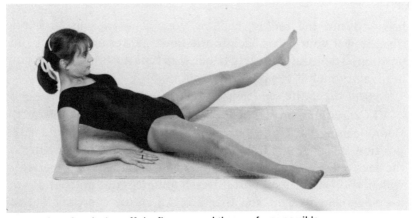

Keeping them four inches off the floor, spread them as far as possible.

cont'd next page

Variations on a Theme (cont'd)

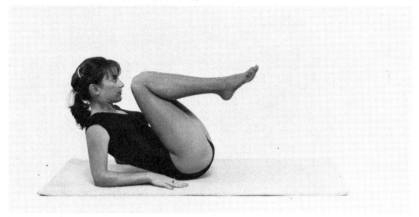

Draw your legs up to your chest, keeping them together.

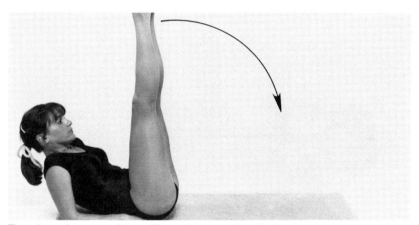

Then shoot them toward the ceiling, hold a second, and bring them back down.

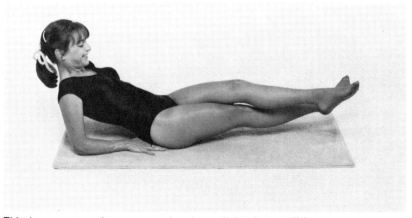

This time, cross your legs, one over the other, still four inches off floor.

cont'd next page

Variations on a Theme (cont'd)

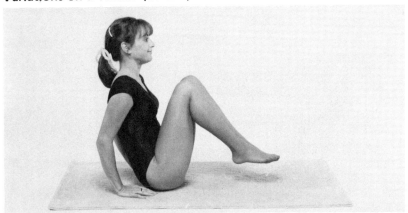
Bring your legs up toward your chest at the same time you raise to a sitting position.

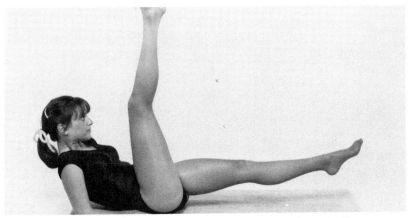
On variation "E" you want to bring your right leg up perpendicular to the floor.

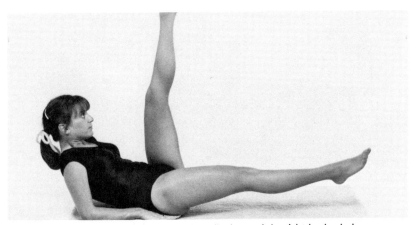
Alternate legs, bringing the left leg up perpendicular, and the right leg back down.

cont'd next page

Variations on a Theme (cont'd)

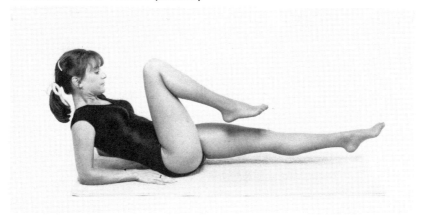

Bring your right leg up toward your chest, keeping your left leg extended.

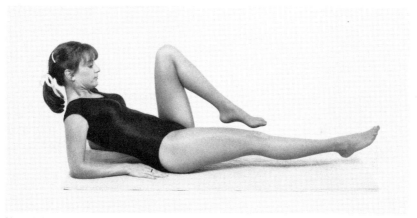

Now, bring your left leg up, while keeping the right leg extended. Alternate.

spread them as you did in "A," and then bring them back toward each other, crossing the right over the left; spread them again; bring them back toward each other, crossing the left over the right; spread them again. Repeat eight times.

D. Starting with your legs straight out in front of you and four inches off the floor, draw your legs to your chest, while you push yourself to a sitting position, and then return them to their starting position. Repeat eight times.

E. Start with your legs extended straight in front of you and four inches off the floor. Keeping your left leg where it is, kick the right leg up (keeping it straight). Bring the right leg down, and as you do, kick the left leg up, allowing them to cross about two feet off the ground in a scissors-like motion. Repeat eight times.

104 KEEPING ALL SYSTEMS FLEXIBLE

F. With both legs extended straight in front of you, and four inches off the ground, draw your right knee to your chest, keeping the left leg straight. Hold for a count of two, and as you return the right leg to its straight position four inches off the floor, bring the left leg up to your chest, so that you are making an exaggerated cycling motion with the legs. Repeat eight times.

Relax a moment, resting your legs on the floor, count to 10, take a deep breath and repeat the entire set of sequences. You should do the entire set four times.

VII. Venus Fly Trap—Lie with your back on the floor, keeping your legs straight and your arms outstretched above your head, as though you were executing a perfect dive into a swimming pool. The exercise is done to the count of five.

On the count of one: Sit up, bringing your outstretched arms over your head so that they are directly in front of you, parallel to the floor; simultaneously, draw your knees to your chest and do not allow your feet to touch the floor.

Count of two: Straighten your legs in front of you, heels on floor.

Count of three: Grasp ankles and touch your nose to your knees while keeping the legs straight.

Count of four: Resume your sitting position, back straight, knees drawn to chest, feet off the floor, and arms outstretched in front of you, parallel to the floor.

Count of five: Conclude by again lying outstretched on the floor.

Repeat sequence 20 times.

Venus Fly Trap

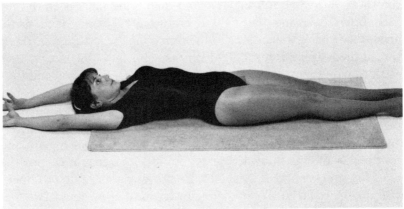

Start in a fully extended position on your back, on your exercise mat.

cont'd next page

Venus Fly Trap (cont'd)

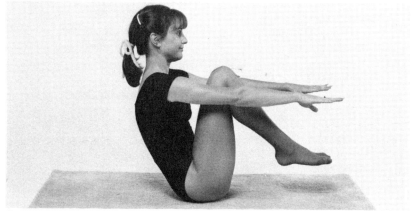

Come up to a sitting position while raising legs to chest and holding out arms.

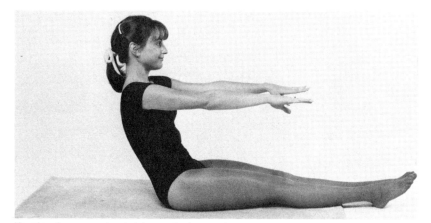

Keeping the arms extended, lower the legs to the mat, keeping them straight.

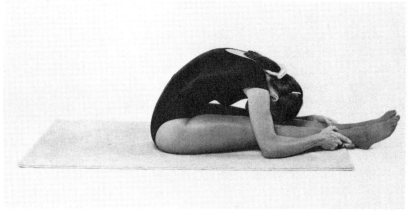

Keeping the legs straight, grasp your ankles and bring your head to your knees.

cont'd next page

Venus Fly Trap (cont'd)

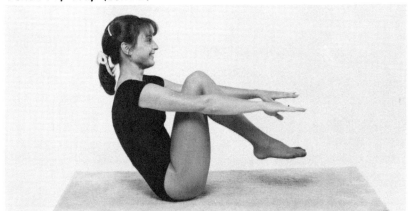

Go back into the sitting position, again with knees to chest and arms out.

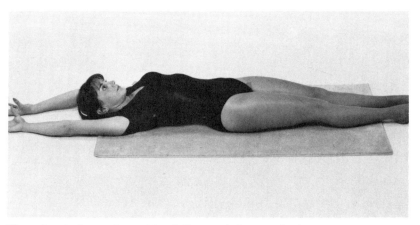

Then return to the starting position, fully extended on your back.

VIII. Piece'o'Pie—Lie on your back, with your legs together and straight and arms outstretched over your head, as in exercise VII. Bring your left foot and right hand together, at a point over your body, creating a pyramid, keeping leg and arm straight. Return to the original position as soon as fingertips touch the foot. Do the same exercise using the left arm and right leg. Repeat the sequence 20 times.

IX. Double-Hand Toe-Touch—Lie on the floor with your legs together and arms outstretched over your head. Assume a sitting position while you simultaneously spread your legs as far as they will comfortably go. Bending at the waist, try to bring your hands down all the way in front of you to the floor, *gently* bouncing

Piece 'O' Pie

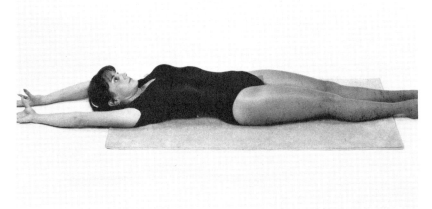

Start in a fully extended position on the floor, on your back.

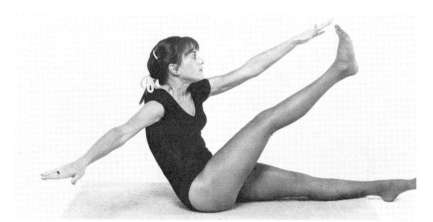

Now alternately come up, touching your left hand to your right foot.

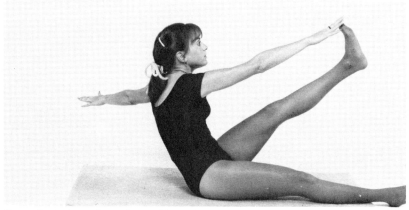

Remember to keep alternating, and keep the arms and legs straight at all times.

twice. Return to a sitting position, arms still raised above your head. Rotate at the waist and bend at the waist to touch your left foot with your outstretched hands, attempting to touch your left ear to your left knee, bouncing gently twice. Resume the sitting position, your arms still outstretched above your head. Rotate at the waist to the right, bending at the waist to touch your right foot with your right hand, attempting to touch your right ear to your right knee, bouncing gently twice. Resume the sitting position, your arms still outstretched above your head. Now, again bend at the waist, coming down onto the floor, touching your hands there, twice bouncing gently before returning to your sitting position. Now, bring your legs together and lie down on the floor, your arms still outstretched as though in a dive. Relax to a count of five, and then repeat the exercise sequence 10 times.

Double-Hand Toe-Touch

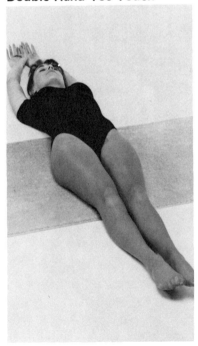

Begin with a fully extended position.

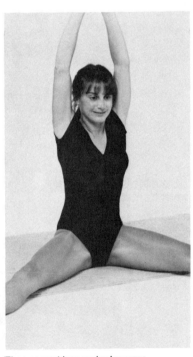

Then spread legs and raise arms.

cont'd next page

Double-Hand Toe-Touch (cont'd)

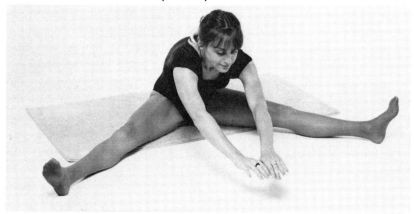

Reach out as far as you can in front of you, keeping legs straight.

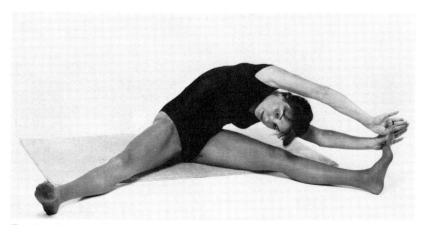

Then bend at the waist to touch your hands to your left leg.

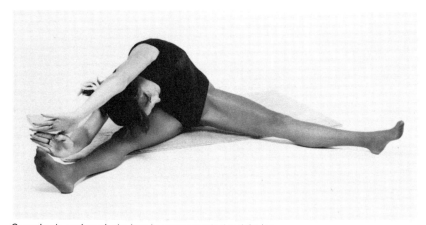

Come back, and reach the hands out to touch the right leg.

110 KEEPING ALL SYSTEMS FLEXIBLE

X. Pelvis Plus—While lying on your back, draw your feet up as close as possible to the buttocks, soles flat on the floor, feet about 12 inches apart. Put your arms out to your sides in order to widen your base and offer support. Raise your pelvis off the floor and keep it up there for the duration of the exercise. Spread your knees apart and then bring them together as though clapping them; repeat eight times. Still keeping the pelvis up, support yourself with your left leg; extend the right leg upward so that it is perpendicular to the floor; now flex your right leg so that your heel approaches your buttocks, then extend the leg so it is parallel to the floor, keeping it straight. Do this combination a total of eight

Pelvis Plus

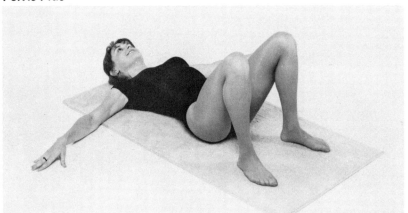

Lie on your back, looking at the ceiling, your arms out, and your feet planted.

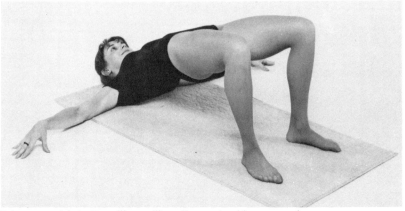

Raise your pelvis to the ceiling, rolling off your shoulders as you do so.

cont'd next page

Pelvis Plus (cont'd)

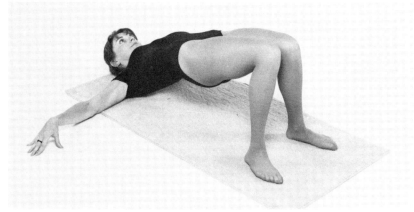

Now bring your knees together, lightly clapping them together.

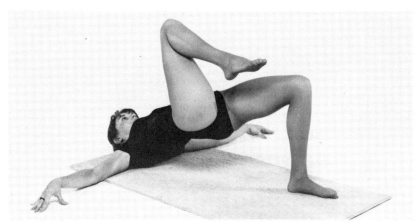

Now bring your right leg off the ground, keeping your leg bent.

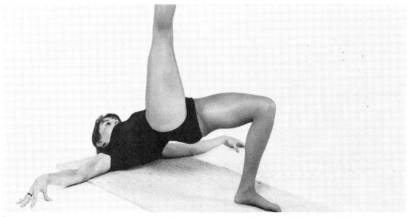

Then raise your leg perpendicular to the floor, keeping it as straight as possible.

cont'd next page

Pelvis Plus (cont'd)

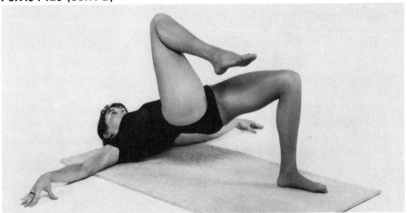

Now bring it back down to a bent position, with your heel going toward your buttocks.

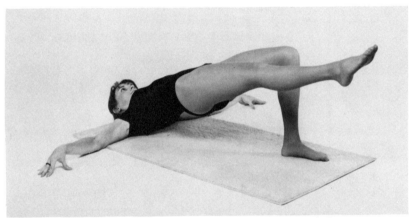

Then extend your leg outward, parallel to the floor, holding it there before return.

times. Bring the right leg down to assume the support of the uplifted pelvis, and repeat the same sequence with the left leg. Return the left leg to the floor behind your buttocks and, with both legs offering support, drop and lift the pelvis eight times. Rest briefly and repeat the sequence three more times.

XI. Crossbones—While lying on your back on the floor, draw your knees up and cross your ankles, striving to spread your knees as far as possible. Place your hands behind your head with your fingers intertwined. Bring your chin up and touch it to your chest, while touching your elbows together in front of your head. Repeat 100 times.

Crossbones

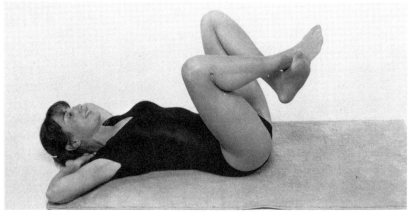

Lie on your back, and cross your ankles, keeping your knees as far apart as possible.

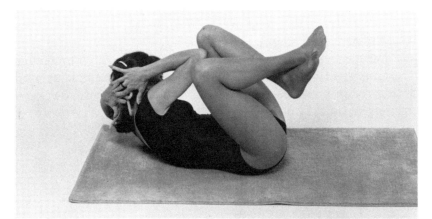

Now alternating touching elbows to opposite knees, start with right elbow to left knee.

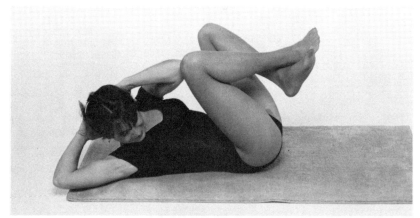

Remember to touch your chin to your chest on each rep and keep the knees spread.

XII. Dog-And-Hydrant—Get down on all fours. Keeping it bent, swing your right leg up to the outside of your body until it is even with the hip. Return it to the floor. Immediately raise your left leg in the same manner. Return it to the original position. Repeat 20 times.

Now swing your bent right leg up to hip level again, your head up and staring forward. Your back should be straight. Now, extend your leg out to the side, keeping it parallel to the floor, and then bring it back. Repeat 20 times. Return to the starting position and do the same with the left leg. Return to the original position and repeat again 20 times with the right leg, and then 20 times with the left leg. Return to your original position.

Pick up your right leg and extend it out to the right, parallel to the floor. Turn your foot to point the toes toward the floor and lower the leg (while keeping it straight) to the floor and return it 20 times. Repeat the same exercise on the left side. Then repeat it on the right side, and again on the left.

Conclude by raising your straightened right leg as far up behind you (and slightly to the side) as it will go. Continue holding your position with your head, your hands and your left leg. Now, bend the right leg at the knee and attempt to touch the right buttock 20 times. Do the same exercise for the left side.

Dog-And-Hydrant

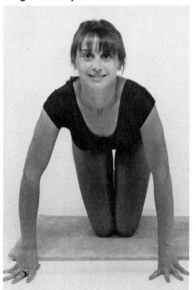

Start this exercise three-quarters of the way across your exercise mat. so you'll have space to touch down with your toes.

cont'd next page

Dog-And-Hydrant (cont'd)

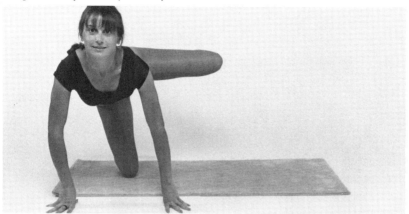

Supporting yourself like a three-legged table, bring the left leg up parallel to floor.

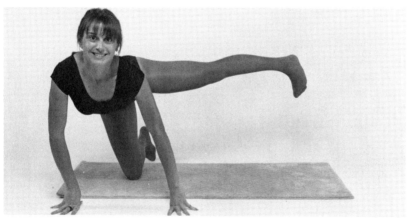

Then extend the leg out, making it straight, but turning the toes downward.

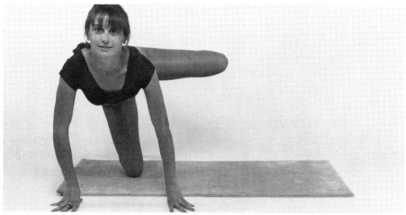

Then bring the leg back into a position where it is bent, heel touching buttocks.

cont'd next page

Dog-And-Hydrant (cont'd)

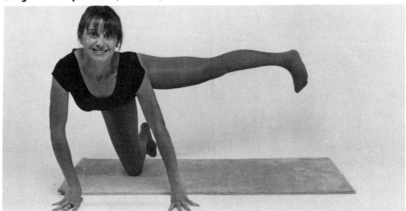

Now extend the leg again, keeping it straight, and again turning toes downward.

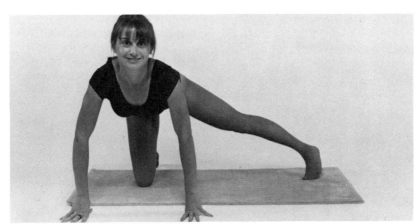

Now gently touch the toes to the floor, keeping your balance and keeping leg straight.

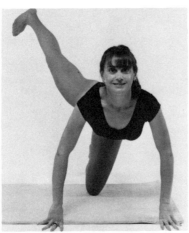

Now extend your leg up and back.

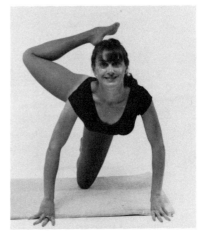

Then bend it to touch buttocks.

XIII. **Skullduggery**—Spread your legs as far apart as they will go while in a standing position, keeping your feet pointed forward. Don't push beyond the sensation of gentle stretching in the groin. Put your arms out straight at your sides, parallel to the ground. Keeping your face up and forward, bend at the waist until the upper portion of your body is parallel to the floor. Bounce *gently* eight times.

Now place your hands behind your back and drop your head, keeping your legs apart. Bounce gently eight times, attempting to touch your head to the floor. Once you do contact the floor, hold in that position for a moment. Raise yourself and return to a nornal standing position. Do this one only on a skid-free surface.

Take a deep breath. Grab a towel and wipe off the perspiration. And hit the showers. You're finished!

Skullduggery

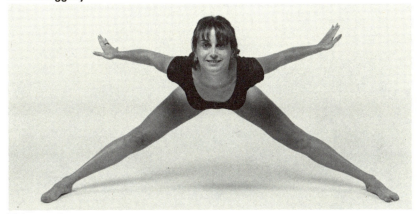

This one takes some practice but it is easier than it looks. Work on balance.

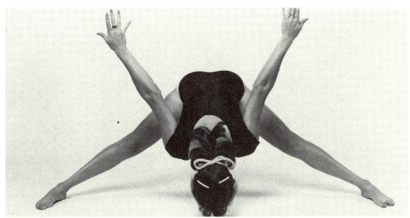

Touch your forehead to the floor in front of you, and then return to starting pose.

4

Spinning Your Wheels
by Richard Benyo

Have you noticed the increasing number of bicyclists lately? We are in the midst of a bicycling revolution that is similar to the running revolution of the late-1970s. Unlike running, however, which is being done purely for sport, bicycling is also being done as an alternative form of vehicular transportation. Additionally, people are cycling because it is fun, and it's good for your health if done regularly and safely. A dedicated following has developed and there are various levels and styles of bicycling just as there are in running. There is a movement now for equal rights with cars to *share* the roads and streets.

In most countries of the world, bicycling has always been accepted as a viable form of transportation, because few countries have a highly industrialized, mobile society like the United States. The Asian countries rely heavily on the bicycle for their survival. Photographs taken by tourists in Red China show millions of people walking and bicycling. Bicycles are everywhere in downtown Peking. In European countries, the bicycle is often used for local jaunts in order to conserve expensive gasoline and racers there have a professional circuit.

In the United States, the automobile has always overshadowed every other form of transportation since its inception. When the motorized vehicle came along, it quickly moved the horse off the roads and took little time in turning the train into a second-rate means of transportation. The bicycle was popular when the automobile took over, but quickly gained toy-status when compared to the automobile. It became a vehicle for having fun, a toy for children. It was not to be considered a vehicle that an adult normally bought and used for the next 60 years.

If you lived in a small town, and if you grew up in the 1950s, you could probably count on one hand the number of adults you saw riding a bicycle. Yet, you'd need a mess of fingers to count the number of your fellow kids who had bicycles. They were everywhere. And everyone knew every other bike in town, so there was no need to lock them. If you left your bicycle outside overnight in the front yard you were likely to get a tongue-lashing from your mother, not because she was afraid someone would steal it, but because she didn't want the dew getting on it and causing rust.

With the new awareness of the benefits of exercise and the weekly rise in gasoline prices, adults are taking to the bicycle in record numbers.

Legions of them can be seen commuting to work on a bicycle when the weather is good. Many are taking 30- and 40-mile weekend rides and the ultimate challenge of the century ride (100 miles) is becoming as popular as running a marathon. Bicycles are being used to run errands, for keeping doctors' appointments, for exercise and frequently by injured runners who want to maintain their level of fitness while they are healing. In a few cities, community employees are being paid mileage if they use their bicycles on the job; in some companies, employees who bicycle to and from work are being given mileage bonuses in their paychecks.
paychecks.

Bicycles offer many practical benefits. They are much easier to maneuver and park than an automobile, and are perfect for doing minor shopping around the neighborhood. But from a fitness standpoint, bicycling is right in there with running and swimming as an excellent aerobic sport. It builds cardiovascular fitness when done regularly. It strengthens the lungs and the heart, and increases the efficiency by which the body uses oxygen. Calories are burned and muscles toned, especially those in the lower body. It builds the hands and strengthens the arms, which are used to support the upper body.

Cycling programs have been recommended for some years as a means of coming back from heart problems—while under the close supervision of a cardiac specialist, of course.

I enjoy taking long Saturday treks on my bicycle, stopping along the way for a picnic lunch that's packed in my knapsack.

There is a certain exhilaration in rolling along a country road at 15 mph, breathing in the early-morning clean air. And when it's early, automobile traffic is still light. You may feel the road was built just for you, of being one with it. The cyclist has an infinitely greater range than someone on foot, and as another cyclist pointed out to me: "When you run, you have to concentrate on running; you can take a drink of water once in a while, but you can't eat or you'll get side stitches. A cyclist though, can eat as much as he wants and it never bothers him." There is a certain feeling of Huckleberry Finn adventure to cycling.

One of the main reasons I purchased my current bicycle, however, was because I was invariably getting injured running in the winter. My legs give out around December, and I'm hobbled for several months. When my next annual running injury came, I was prepared and took to the bicycle, quadrupling my mileage (about four bicycling miles equal one running mile in training benefits if both are done on level ground), and managed to keep my fitness level up pretty well. As the injury began healing, I would pedal my bicycle a few miles to get the leg warmed up, go by the local dirt running track, put in a few laps, and hop back on the bike to get home, using the ride home to cool down from the workout. It brought me back from my injury much faster than I'd come back in previous years. Of course, having become interested in cycling for the first time since childhood, I was reluctant to give it up just because I was healed enough to run again. So as April rolled around, I went on a 50-mile bicycle trip through Northern California's Napa Valley wine country. At mile 47, I hit some railroad tracks that were diagonal to the road, got my front wheel stuck and went over the handlebars, breaking my bike, my camera, my glasses and my collarbone (I don't recall in which order). The injury effectively kept me from running or cycling for a few weeks in my annual spring attempt to get into competitive shape. My cycling had done what my annual winter injury had pretty much failed to do—stop me cold in my tracks.

I was kind of a clumsy bike rider as a kid, and I'd managed to continue being clumsy as an adult. Although some people can ride bicycles without using their hands, take turns by leaning their bodies and flow smoothly with automobile traffic during rush hour, I'm pretty much a wreck looking for a place to hang it up. As exhilarating as it is to roll along a deserted country road at 8:00 Saturday morning, it is equally (but conversely) as frightening to try to ride a bicycle in traffic.

Which brings me, in a roundabout way, to the subject of stationary, indoor bicycles. They can be ridden without fear of being struck by a car. A stationary bike is exactly what it sounds like—a bicycle that you pedal, but that goes nowhere. It's the only bicycle I've been able to ride without hands. (Another benefit: it doesn't get flats.)

The most elemental of the stationary bicycles uses parts of a regular bicycle, usually ignoring the rear wheel and holding the whole apparatus to a stand that can often be anchored to the floor by bolts—if you want to go that far. Rather than the drive train going to the rear wheel, though, the chain connects with the front wheel and turns it. The handlebars are fixed (but can usually be adjusted up or down for the rider's comfort) and the seat is more comfortable than 10-speed bicycles feature; the seat, too, is usually adjustable. Stationary bicycles can be bought assembled or in pieces.

Many novice exercisers buy a device such as a stationary bicycle and enjoy it for a few days, but then burn themselves out on it, and shove it into a dark corner of the garage. The stationary bicycle is not difficult to store in most cases, but the more sophisticated a bike you buy, the more awkward it usually is, and the more difficult it is to push off into a corner. It wants attention. After all, it was paid for with perfectly good money.

For those who have become obsessed with gym equipment, the bicycle has a way of winding up as part of the living room furniture. I've known people who take every opportunity to use their exercise bicycle. They'll read a book while pumping, watch their favorite television shows, compose songs, or go into a trance state. They leave their bicycles parked in the middle of the living room 24 hours a day. Visitors must talk around the stationary bicycle no matter where they sit in the room.

When it comes to an assistant in the quest for fitness, the stationary bicycle is one of the most economical, easy-to-use and easy-to-understand devices, which might be why there are so many fanatics. And almost everyone has ridden a bicycle at some time during his life, so jumping onto an exercise cycle and pedaling off to nowhere is easy. The secret to not burning out is caution, patience and starting your program from a logical point. Just because you rode a bicycle when you were 16, doesn't mean that at a sedentary 36 you can jump onto the new exercise cycle and act as though you're trying out for a starring role in *"Breaking Away, Part II."*

Neither does your seriousness in beginning an indoor exercise program mean that you have to rush out and purchase a top-of-the-line stationary cycle. You needn't pay a lot of money to prove that you are serious about getting into fitness in a big way. The monkey-hide seats are swell, but not really conducive to fitness, and the coon tail on an antenna with a fan mounted on the handlebars to make it stream back behind you even though you are still stationary is a useless gesture unless you also buy the helmet and goggles to keep the wind out of your eyes.

If you are not grossly overweight (and you shouldn't be if you are getting into advanced forms of exercise), almost any good stationary bicycle will serve the needed functions—if it is taken care of, maintained properly and is not abused by being allowed to sit out in the rain for a month.

In the basic stationary bicycle look for the following signs of quality:

1. Solid construction. Give the store's demonstration model a good shake; if it rattles or something is threatening to fall off don't buy it. Check the welding to make sure it is consistent and capable of holding your weight.

2. Good warranty and service. Make sure that the store from which you purchase your exercise cycle can service it, and be sure there is a manufacturer's warranty. If there is none don't buy it. If there is a full warranty, how long does it last? If it is a limited warranty, what is it limited to? And, on the limited warranty, if you are responsible for certain parts or certain labor charges, what are they expected to be for normal breakdowns or regular maintenance?

3. Ease of maintenance. Inquire if regular maintenance, such as oiling the chain or taking up slack in the friction devices on the wheel (usually standard bicycle hand brakes), must be done at the store where you bought it, or if it can be done quickly and easily at home.

4. Stability. Riding the demonstration model, slowly build up speed. Is the base solid enough or does it begin to vibrate and sway when the speed increases? How is the foundation built? Will it scar the surface of your living room if you intend to use it there? Will you need to put a throw-rug or a canvas tarp under it? Does it have wheels attached for ease of movement? How long has the manufacturer been doing business and what other fitness apparatus or hardware does the company make?

5. Good, easy-to-read instructions. Most stationary bicycles feature instruments that show speed, your mileage and a pre-set timer. Some of the instruments fall apart or go haywire on their way home from the store; others are so rugged and effective they look as though they were part of a manufacturer's overrun for the NASA space shuttle. The instruments should be of good quality and should be mentioned specifically in the warranty agreement. Give the instruments a rap with your knuckle; if they rattle or sound the least bit frail, forget that cycle, because they'll be getting a grueling workout.

6. Reliable, well-established dealer. Try to buy from a dealer who has been around for a while and who you feel you can go back to if you need help either in understanding the machine further or in getting repairs and accessories. The dealer is usually your link to the manufacturer, and he can be one of your best allies or worst enemies.

7. Adjustability. Not everyone is the same size, weight, has the same length of arms and legs, etc. To compensate for the differences an exercise bicycle should be completely adjustable. See that you can set the handlebars and the seat to your individual needs. Some exercise cycles allow the use of different seats (although the unit comes with only one seat). That's because many use the same seat post design found on most 10-speed bicycles. Let's face it, not everyone's fanny is going to be equally as comfortable on a standard seat. You may want to try the anatomically designed Avocet seat. (Bicycle seats, by the way, are also referred to as "saddles.") The seat should be adjusted so that at the bottom of the pedal thrust, your knee is still bent a bit; don't set the seat so high that your leg is straight at the bottom of the thrust. If you do, your knee is going to feel a strain, and so will your Achilles tendon.

TWO VARIATIONS ON A THEME

For this chapter, we are going to use two machines and two exercise programs, one for each of the units. One exercise cycle is quite basic, while the other is more complex. Although the design of the second machine is more sophisticated and works more parts of the body, it is equally easy to use.

THE BASIC EXERCISE CYCLE

The simplest exercise cycle imaginable would be a one-speed

bicycle, with hand brakes, that is mounted on rollers and supported so that the rider does not have to balance. In order to approximate outdoor conditions, the front rollers could be raised to create a hill.

Although most companies do not use standard bicycle frames, the frames are very much the same. The basic exercise cycle looks like a stunted bicycle. It is mounted on a stand and has no rear wheel. The handlebars are recognizable, and so are the pedals and the seat. The power (usually through a standard bicycle chain) is fed to the front wheel, which spins. The front wheel features adjustable brakes or some other device that causes rolling resistance, and makes pedaling more difficult. The unit almost always features a speedometer and an odometer.

The unit we've been using is a very compact model, called the Marcy Bodycycle. It features a spring that tightens a belt around the wheel, and is adjustable from a panel down between the handlebars. There is a numbered scale to indicate the range of effort you can set into the machine; the resistance can be adjusted while you are riding the machine, by leaning down and screwing the adjustment to a new setting.

As with any machine (from a food processor to an automobile to the space shuttle), you should familiarize yourself with its design before using it. Get on the seat and try the variable-resistance knob. Pedal at different speeds. You'll soon become comfortable with the exercise cycle and will be in no way intimidated or awed by it.

Sit on the cycle and get comfortable. Check the seat height. If your leg, extended down toward the floor, while your heel is on the pedal, cannot flex just slightly at the knee, at the longest part of the stroke, the seat is too high; if your leg bends excessively at the knee, the seat is too low.

Start using the machine at its lowest-possible resistance setting. Just pedal a minute or two to get the feel of it. You will tend to pump it fast at first. Pedal gently and slowly to get a feel for the pedals and for balancing on your seat. Don't go into a racing crouch when you first hop onto the machine, turning the pedals at 90 rpm. Begin gently, giving your legs a chance to warm up, and then build your speed gradually. This will minimize leg soreness and injuries.

So play around with the cycle at first; get to know its workings before training on it.

Now that you are familiar with the machine, let's go through a few basic workouts on it and then set up a program.

ROUND ONE

Set the machine at its lowest setting, so that there is virtually no resistance. If your cycle has a timer, set it for five minutes. Now, moving into the pedaling very easily, begin counting to yourself, trying to approximate one complete revolution of the pedals each two seconds, so that you are doing 30 rpm. This will seem too easy and you'll probably, by the end of the first minute, be frustrated with the slow pace. But hold yourself back. Don't push it. Hold that pace for the full five minutes. When the five minutes is up, dismount and take a short walk around the room. Keep walking for at least wo minutes, to get your legs loose.

Then, remount the machine, again set it for five minutes, and do one revolution every second, so that you are doing 60 rpm. When you are finished, dismount, again walk around the room for two minutes, and remount the bike. Set it for five minutes again, drop your speed to 30 rpm as a cool down, and when you are done, walk around for another two minutes. Finish up with a few leg stretches, being careful to do them slowly and gently.

ROUND TWO

That exercise probably seemed almost too tame, but it served two purposes: to get you familiar with the machine and to acquaint you with the principles of warm up, and cool down. The warmup and cooldown are as important as the actual effort period. As you progress, you will keep the warm-up periods fairly standard, but you will significantly expand the effort portion of the routine. Look at exercising like you would a sandwich. You have just done exercise equal to a single slice of cheese placed between two pieces of bread. No matter what you add to the sandwich to enhance it, you'll still have the ingredients enclosed by the two pieces of bread, even if the ingredients begin to form a submarine sandwich.

The object now is to add some resistance.

Your next training session should come two days later. You should not embark on a program of fitness too quickly. This time, set the resistance at the first mark. On the Marcy Bodycycle, it is a "1." The unit goes up to "10," at which point it is almost impossible to turn the darn thing even if you stand up on the pedals with an elephant on your back. Now, do the same workout you did two days ago: five minutes of 30 rpm, followed by walking around for a minute or two, then five minutes of 60 rpm, followed by some more walking around, and then five more minutes of 30 rpm work, and another walk, with some casual stretching worked in.

You'll notice that the effort required to do today's workout was significantly more than the effort required two days ago. If you have a limited amount of time in which to exercise, the resistance control will become your closest ally, because it will allow you to standardize your exercise time while regulating your output.

It is imperative that you do not increase your workload too quickly. Your incredibly adaptable human body will respond to the training, certainly, but it needs sufficient time to make the change safely. Be gentle with yourself; the theory that if it doesn't hurt, it isn't helping, is a myth.

If you are patient, you can keep your effort at an almost-comfortable level and still make progress.

Give yourself a day off following your effort at "1." This is an adaptation of the hard/easy theory of training, in which you put out an effort one day, and allow your body to recuperate from the work the next day. As you progress, the "easy" day will go from one without exercise to one with easy exercise.

For your next work day, let's work a little further with the same machine by doing your warmup at 30 rpm for five minutes, at a setting of "1," followed by some walking. Remount and put the setting to "1.5," and go 60 rpm for five minutes, followed by more walking and then five minutes of 30 rpm at a "1" setting. Finish with some walking and stretching.

Exercise cycles build up the legs, very much like regular bicycles do. There are handles on the exercise cycles, but they are present almost exclusively for support and balance. There is very little benefit to the arms and upper body in bicycling and when using an exercise cycle, except that from supporting some of your weight on your arms. While you gain cardiovascular and leg conditioning, you should consider the entire body in order to maintain a balance of the systems. For upper body work, refer to Chapter 6 where programs on machines and weights that are particularly suited to increasing the strength in the upper body are discussed. As an aside, it has been found that in running, some 10 percent of your power and efficiency can come from the arms, even though they are not directly involved in locomotion. My own findings have been that in the latter stages of a marathon, or in doing hillwork, using my arms when my upper legs begin to tire has great benefits toward keeping myself going strong.

ROUND THREE

Now that you are familiar with the cycle, let's set up a program that will strengthen you gradually. We'll assume that you have no more than a half-hour in which to exercise. And that you do not want to exercise more than five days a week. And that you are not interested in going too far beyond good fitness and into what amounts to competition against your own limits. For those more competitive types, we have the second half of this chapter, which will warm the cockles of their rapidly strengthening hearts. So, let's run down several weeks of training:

Day 01: 5 min 30 rpm at 0, 2 min walk, 5 min 60 rpm at 0, 2 min walk, 5 min 30 rpm at 0, 2 min walk/stretch.

Day 02: rest.

Day 03: 5 min 30 rpm at 1, 2 min walk, 5 min 60 rpm at 1, 2 min walk, 5 min 30 rpm at 1, 2 min walk/stretch.

Day 04: rest.

Day 05: 5 min 30 rpm at 1, 2 min walk, 5 min 60 rpm at 1.5, 2 min walk, 5 min 30 rpm at 1, 2 min walk/stretch.

Day 06: rest.

Day 07: 5 min 30 rpm at 1, 2 min walk, 5 min 60 rpm at 1, 2 min walk, 5 min 30 rpm at 1, 2 min walk/stretch.

Day 08: rest.

Day 09: 5 min 30 rpm at 1, 2 min walk, 5 min 60 rpm at 2, 2 min walk, 5 min 30 rpm at 1, 2 min walk/stretch.

Day 10: rest.

Day 11: 5 min 30 rpm at 1, 2 min walk, 5 min 60 rpm at 2, 2 min walk, 5 min 30 rpm at 1, 2 min walk/stretch.

Day 12: 5 min 30 rpm at 0, 2 min walk, 5 min 60 rpm at 1, 2 min walk, 5 min 30 rpm at 0, 2 min walk/stretch.

Day 13: rest.

Day 14: 5 min 30 rpm at 1, 2 min walk, 7 min 60 rpm at 2, 2 min walk, 5 min 30 rpm at 1, 2 min walk/stretch.

Day 15: 5 min 30 rpm at 0, 2 min walk, 5 min 60 rpm at 1, 2 min walk, 5 min 30 rpm at 0, 2 min walk/stretch.

Day 16: rest.

Day 17: 5 min 30 rpm at 1, 2 min walk, 5 min 60 rpm at 2,5, 2 min walk, 5 min 30 rpm at 1, 2 min walk/stretch.

Day 18: 5 min 30 rpm at 0, 2 min walk, 5 min 60 rpm at 1, 2 min walk, 5 min 30 rpm at 0, 2 min walk/stretch.

Day 19: rest.

Day 20: 5 min 30 rpm at 1, 2 min walk, 5 min 60 rpm at 2.5, 2 min walk, 5 min 30 rpm at 1, 2 min walk/stretch.

Day 21: 5 min 30 rpm at 0, 2 min walk, 7 min 60 rpm at 1, 2 min walk, 5 min 30 rpm at 0, 2 min walk/stretch.

Day 22: rest.

Day 23: 5 min 30 rpm at 1.5, 2 min walk, 7 min 60 rpm at 2.5, 2 min walk, 5 min 30 rpm at 1, 2 min walk/stretch.

Day 24: 5 min 30 rpm at 1, 2 min walk, 5 min 60 rpm at 1.5, 2 min walk, 5 min 30 rpm at 0, 2 min walk/stretch.

Day 25: rest.

Day 26: 5 min 30 rpm at 1.5, 2 min walk, 5 min 60 rpm at 3, 2 min walk, 5 min 30 rpm at 1, 2 min walk/stretch.

Day 27: 5 min 30 rpm at 1, 2 min walk, 5 min 60 rpm at 1.5, 2 min walk, 5 min 30 rpm at 1, 2 min walk/stretch.

Day 28: rest.

Day 29: 5 min 30 rpm at 1.5, 2 min walk, 7 min 60 rpm at 3, 2 min walk, 5 min 30 rpm at 1, 2 min walk/stretch.

Day 30: 5 min 30 rpm at 1, 2 min walk, 5 min 60 rpm at 1.5, 2 min walk, 5 min 30 rpm at 1, 2 min walk/stretch.

Day 31: rest.

To continue progress at a faster rate, it is necessary to continue adding to the intensity of the workouts on a regular basis. You should always remember that the process of exercising (and this reminder will be repeated each chapter) is one of stress and recuperation. You push your body beyond what it is currently capable of and then you fall back to a "rest" period for recovery. Notice in the foregoing schedule that after each strenuous workout there is an easy one, and then a rest day. The easy workout serves as a partial rest day (relative to the hard day), and the rest day is imperative.

If, during the workouts, you begin to feel unusual stress in a specific part of the body (i.e., the Achilles tendon), back off immediately by reducing the workout and schedule a rest day the following day. The day after your rest day try an easier workout than was scheduled. You want to keep the tendon flexible, but not stressed.

If you're feeling lackadaisical, it is probably a reaction to the workouts. Get more sleep, but don't necessarily back off on your workouts. Runners often experience lackluster days several weeks before running a marathon, when they are doing two workouts a day and long mileage. But when they begin their training run, they come alive. Fatigue is merely the body's way of saying, "Hey, I put in a good day's work, between my job and that workout, and I'm signaling you that I want to go to bed and repair myself."

With the basic exercise cycle, such as the Marcy Bodycycle, you can work toward a fitness plateau and once reached hold it there with a regular series of workouts. Perhaps the workout at the twenty-ninth day is enough for you; if it is, so be it. Holding at that level keeps your time investment reasonable and you'll enjoy being fit.

If you want to become ambitious, pushing your fitness to the level where it becomes a game and a challenge, trade in your basic exercise cycle on something more elaborate, like the original Exercycle. It works both the upper and lower body, and has been a standard in the industry for perhaps 40 years. Some of the original units are reputedly still in operation, and the current units have not been changed substantially. It is basically like riding a horse at a gallop: the foot pedals turn and the handlebars move forward and back, giving your upper body a workout and taking it through a wide range of motion.

Schwinn also has a unit available that works both upper and lower body and is called the Air-Dyne. The next set of programs is based on this unit. Before that, however, a few final words of caution on the basic exercise cycle:

Too many people want to become fit too fast, which is only natural, but in the process they do too much too soon. The resulting injuries and exhaustion usually turn them off to exercise in general. Exercise should be a very positive factor in your life; it should be something you look forward to because besides getting immediate good results (a certain liveliness in your step immediately following it), it provides long-term results that stay with you

24 hours a day. Approach exercise as you would approach a friendship that you want to last: allow it to develop, but don't push it. Your body is anxious to cooperate with your exercise plans, but it isn't a rubberband that can be stretched to the limit at a moment's notice. You'll be surprised, however, at just how far it will stretch to accommodate your goals.

GETTING ABOARD BIG GOLD

When they delivered the Schwinn Air-Dyne Exerciser AD-2, a woman from the company came by the very next day to tell me all about it. This is not standard procedure, of course. Since I was going to develop some programs for the cycle and tell you about it, they wanted to make sure I knew its unique characteristics. The saleswoman made an interesting point about indoor exercises that I have ignored. We were discussing the advantages of indoor exercising, especially the ability to get the benefits of bicycling without being run over by a truck. "The thing I like about using an exercise cycle," she said, "is that you can stay inside when the pollution outside is bad. And pollution is always worse outside. Health authorities always tell you to stay inside during a pollution alert in the big cities, so when pollution gets bad, you can still be doing good things for your body by pedaling inside on your cycle,"

That's true. Air pollution had been the least of my concerns because my inclination is to think of the benefits of exercising indoors in terms of saving my life from traffic, muggers, potholes, and various other dangers. I'm also inclined to view its benefits against the elements; when it's raining, you can exercise dry (except for your perspiration); when it's snowing and icy outside, you can work out with no danger greater than rug-burn.

Her point about pollution makes an awful lot of sense, of course, and has significant implications for older people who like to exercise but have to put off exercising when the pollution level becomes intolerable. While pollution vividly affects people who are older and who have had heart or respiratory problems. it affects anyone who is out there breathing it. At one point I thought about writing a novel about a guy who was training for the 1984 Los Angeles Olympic Games. I had him training next to freeways so that he would become accustomed to Los Angeles' smog. Pollution's effect on healthy people is unseen, yet insidious. If you are an exerciser, especially a runner, you can feel your body expending extra effort on a polluted day to get the same amount of work

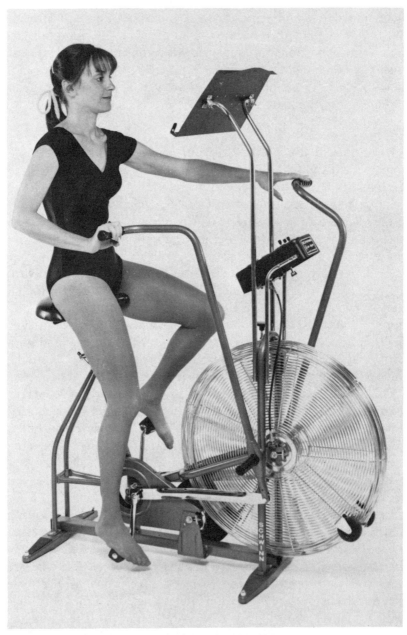

The Air Dyne unit exercises the arms and legs simultaneously, while producing a flow of cooling air.

Spinning Your Wheels 133

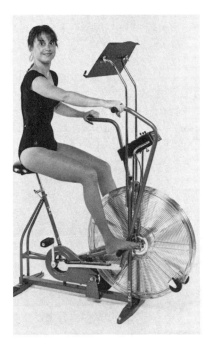

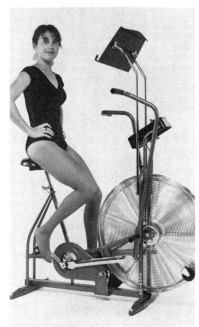

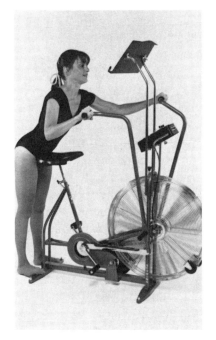

The Air Dyne unit can be used as only a cycling machine (upper left) by using only the foot pedals, since the handles for exercising the arms are integrated with the foot pedals. Conversely, the machine provides bars (upper right) on which you can rest your feet while using only the upper body exercising feature. The handles can also be used effectively from a slightly different angle by standing behind the machine (left) and pumping.

accomplished on the last cool, clear day. There won't be any world record set in the 1500 meters at the Los Angeles Olympic Games; you can make book on that.

Although the ocean winds and fog make it rare to find a really polluted day in the San Francisco Bay Area, there are occasions when the winds forget to blow, the temperature rises and with no place to go the foul air hangs around like bad breath. I had the Air-Dyne set up in the warehouse at our office, and wouldn't you know it, the first day I used it was a day with mustard-colored air. The words of the Schwinn saleswoman made a lot of sense, so what I did was go to the local racquetball blub, change into my running clothes, run the two miles to the office, use the Air-Dyne in the warehouse, and then run two miles back to the racquetball club, where I showered and then returned to work.

I felt tired running to work in the dirty air. Once inside the air-conditioned offices, however, I revived quickly and enjoyed examining the Air-Dyne up close.

Excelsior Fitness Equipment Company, an adjunct of Schwinn, the bicycle maker, markets the exercise cycle. The unit is quite unique in that resistance is created in wind vanes (instead of through brake friction) and it features handles integrated with the pedals that work the upper body at the same time as the legs. The handles can be used independently of the pedals. Introduced in the fall of 1978, the unit is advertised as being a combination of the best benefits of a rowing machine and a conventional exercise bicycle. The exercise cycle features wheels attached to the front of the fully enclosed vanes that make it easy to tilt forward and move around. There is a safety lock for the moving parts in case you happen to be in possession of one or more curious children, and the seat is fully adjustable. It can be removed so that you can put on any seat you want to use. There is a device that measures the amount of ergometric exercise you are getting; the faster you work the unit, the more resistance is offered. The wind vane feature has an interesting side effect: as you are exercising to turn it, it is providing a cool breeze, something no other exercise cycle features. The price of the unit as of August 1981 was $495.

Before mounting the Air-Dyne, let's take a look at something of interest to those who are disciples of Dr. Ken Cooper. In his books (*Aerobics, The Aerobics Way*, etc.) he advocates for people to exercise regularly in sports and activities that emphasize aerobics. "Aerobics" means "with air." The opposite or converse of

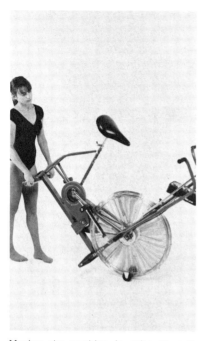
Moving the machine is quite easy; it features convenient wheels on front.

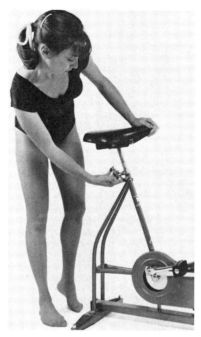
As with a bicycle, seat adjustment is important—and making the adjustment is easy.

"aerobics" is "anaerobic," or "without air." If you are a reasonably healthy person you may take a brisk walk and though your breathing increases, you are still functioning at an aerobic level; if, as you are walking along in that brisk shuffle, you see a friend crossing the street some blocks away and you break into a sprint to try and catch him before he vanishes, you are likely to push yourself beyond *your* "aerobic threshold" into anaerobic. Your breathing becomes labored and you are gasping for air. There is a fine line between aerobic and anaerobic, and that threshold is the basis of all endurance sports. In a long-distance runner's training, the idea is to become so efficient at the aerobic level that the aerobic threshold is constantly being increased, so that it takes more and more effort to go into anaerobic.

Pushing the aerobic threshold back builds up your cardiorespiratory system: that integrated system between your body's intake of oxygen and the bloodstream's ability to move the oxygen to your muscles in order to keep them working. Such exercise also strengthens the heart. Dr. Cooper further states that aerobic workouts done on a regular basis reduce the risk of heart disease.

Ken Cooper has quantified how much aerobic exercise must be done each week to experience its highly beneficial effect. His system gives points for however much exercise is done. A list of points and exercises is provided to compare different sports. If you can amass 30 of Ken Cooper's aerobic points a week, you will enjoy the benefits of aerobic exercise and protect yourself against heart disease. (People who train for marathons and other like endurance events go far beyond Cooper's point system. But anything beyond 30 points is just for your own benefit. You may even be risking fatigue with so much exercise. Therefore, in a two-hour run while in training for a marathon, the first 20 - 30 minutes is for your health, and the rest is for your head.

A chart has been worked out for the Schwinn ergoMet™ Exerciser (a.k.a. Air-Dyne) that corresponds to Cooper's points system. It is reproduced below:

AEROBIC POINTS PER TWELVE MINUTES OF EXERCISE USING

ergoMetric™ Exerciser Workload Settings

Body-weight (lbs)	0.5	1.0	1.5	2.0	2.5	3.0	3.5	4.0	5.0	6.0	7.0
77-99	1.1	2.6	4.4	7.1	10.8	15.3	20.8	—	—	—	—
100-121	.7	1.7	2.9	4.4	6.5	9.4	12.5	16.4	—	—	—
122-143	.5	1.1	1.5	3.1	4.4	6.1	8.3	10.8	17.1	—	—
144-165	—	.9	1.1	2.4	3.2	4.4	5.9	7.5	11.9	17.4	—
166-187	—	.5	.9	1.9	2.6	3.3	4.4	5.7	8.8	13.1	18.4
188-209	—	—	.8	1.4	2.1	2.8	3.4	4.4	6.7	10.0	13.7
210-231	—	—	.6	1.1	1.7	2.3	2.9	3.5	5.3	7.8	10.8
232-253	—	—	.5	1.0	1.4	1.9	2.5	3.0	4.3	6.3	8.8
254-275	—	—	—	.8	1.1	1.6	2.1	2.6	3.6	5.2	7.1

The chart works off a 12-minute exercise session. The numbers running across the top of the chart are the levels of effort being expended and are calibrated on a gauge on the machine. The numbers down the left column are the weight divisions for you. So, if you weigh 155 pounds and you go 12 minutes at a 2.5 effort, you have amassed 3.2 of Cooper's aerobic points, and all you need for the remainder of the week is 26.8 points. If you are just starting to use something like the Air-Dyne, you'll start at the easier levels and work your way up as you become stronger and as your cardiovascular (or cardiorespiratory) system develops.

This is a good time, before we get right into pumping away on the cycle, to look at oxygen use, calories burned for an activity, and so on. We love to measure what we're doing in order to know how well we are performing or what benefit it is bringing us. The following chart breaks down into three segments. The middle segment is the basis of the chart; it includes information on the expenditure of energy of a hypothetical individual. Forget about the oxygen uptake. You remember our discussion of mets in the first chapter; a met is an arbitrary measurement of work based on your sitting around doing absolutely nothing, which translates into 1 met. Get up and go to the refrigerator for a beer and you're increasing your mets. The more mets you use, the more calories you burn. You burn calories sitting around doing nothing because you need energy (and energy is produced by burning calories) just to breathe and for your body to function. Increase your mets use and your calorie use also increases, which is the whole basis of weight loss through exercise.

Now look at the left and right segments. One refers to a bicycle ergometer and the other refers to running on a treadmill (one capable of increasing its grade, as in Chapter 2).

You needn't become concerned about interpreting all of the nuances of the numbers. The chart is reproduced specifically to show you the direct relationships that are in effect when you exercise on a piece of indoor exercise equipment. The three calories you're burning at 2.4 mets while walking at two miles per hour on a level treadmill is comparable to 150 kpm/min on the bicycle ergometer.

Increase your mets to 5.0 and you are burning six calories. To raise your work effort to 5.0 mets you can either be walking at 3 mph on the treadmill with it set at a 5 percent grade, or you can be putting out 450 kpm/min. on the bicycle ergometer and accomplish the same.

Naturally, the harder you push on this, or the more calories you burn, the more benefits to your cardiorespiratory system and

OXYGEN COST OF VARIOUS BICYCLE ERGOMETER AND TREADMILL WORKLOADS

Bicycle Ergometer External Work Output		Energy Expenditure of an Average individual (70 kg body weight)	
(kpm/min*)	(watts†)	Total O_2 Uptake (liters/min)	O_2 Uptake (ml/kg/min)
150	25	0.6	8.5
300	50	0.9	13.0
450	75	1.2	17.0
600	100	1.5	21.0
750	125	1.8	26.0
900	150	2.1	30.0
1050	175	2.4	36.0
1200	200	2.7	39.0
1350	225	3.0	43.0
1500	250	3.3	47.0
1650	275	3.6	51.0
1800	300	3.9	56.0

*Kilopond-meter: Energy necessary to lift a 1-kg mass 1 meter against the normal gravitational force.
†Watt: A unit of power equal to 6.12 kpm/min.

OXYGEN COST OF VARIOUS BICYCLE ERGOMETER AND TREADMILL WORKLOADS (CONT.)

Energy Expenditure of an Average individual (70 kg body weight) (CONT.)		Treadmill (3 minutes at each level to achieve a steady state)	
Mets‡	Calories** (per min)	Speed (mph)	Grade (%)
2.4	3.0	2.0	0.0
3.7	4.5	3.0	0.0
5.0	6.0	3.0	5.0
6.0	7.5	3.0	7.5
7.0	9.0	3.0	10.0
8.5	10.5	3.0	15.0
10.0	12.0	4.0	10.0
11.0	14.0	4.0	14.0
12.0	15.0	7.0 (running)	0.0
		3.5	16.0
13.5	17.0	4.0	18.0
14.5	13.0	3.5	20.0
16.0	20.0	8.0 (running)	0.0
		4.2	16.0
		3.5	26.0
		4.0	22.0
		10.0 (running)	0.0
		5.0	18.0

‡Met: Basal O_2 requirement of the body in an inactive state, sitting quietly. Considered by most authorities to be 3.5 ml O_2/kg/min.
**Calorie: A unit of energy based on heat production. One calorie equals 200 ml of O_2 consumed.

to your muscle groups—to a point. You should not enter such programs, however, with an attitude that you can move down the chart within a week or two. Start at a level that is comfortable and gradually improve at a regular, but careful speed.

There is a tendency, especially among people who are competitive by nature, to look at such a chart and want to run right off the end of it by out-performing the machine. Remember my own experiences with the treadmill test in Chapter 1; unless there is a power failure or a mechanical breakdown, the machine is always capable of going longer.

Too many people who embark on an exercise program do so demanding immediate results from it. This is both dangerous and unrealistic. An exercise program should begin carefully. If you have been away from exercise for some time, expect to see slow, steady progress rather than huge accomplishments.

Many people wake up one dreary morning, look in the mirror and don't like what they see they've become. They decide to do something about recapturing that beautiful body from the past. So they join health clubs or buy exercise bicycles for the home and spend hours at a time working themselves silly, sweating like bulls in heat, huffing and puffing, and generally becoming overbearing pains in the ass. Too much exercise too soon for these out-of-shape people creates ogres who moan and groan a lot and demand sympathy. After a week of being unable to get out of bed without assistance and turning off everyone they come in contact with, the mad exercisers once again present themselves to their mirrors and learn that there has been no magic alteration. These people usually let the exercise bicycle gather dust in a corner of the garage and spend the rest of their lives going around bad-mouthing exercise.

Exercise for the beginner should be like learning sword swallowing. Take your time, relax, ease into it gently, and don't try to swallow the whole thing the first week. The consequences are too tragic to think about.

There's one more chart I'd like to share with you. I've found it fascinating because it expands on the chart that has gone before, and puts many occupational and recreational pursuits into focus because it groups them side-by-side on the same line with the strict scientific information about mets, oxygen uptake and calories being burned. This chart comes from the American Heart Association.

APPROXIMATE METABOLIC COST OF ACTIVITIES*

	Occupational	Recreational
1½–2 METs† 4–7 ml O_2/min/kg 2–2½ kcal/min (70 kg person)	Desk work Auto driving ‡ Typing Electric calculating machine operation	Standing Walking (strolling 1.6 km or 1 mile/hr) Flying, motorcycling ‡ Playing cards ‡ Sewing, knitting
2–3 METs 7–11 ml O_2/min/kg 2½–4 kcal/min (70 kg person)	Auto repair Radio, TV repair Janitorial work Typing, manual Bartending	Level walking (3.2 km or 2 miles/hr) Level bicycling (8.0 km or 5 miles/hr) Riding lawn mower Billiards, bowling Skeet shuffleboard Woodworking (light) Powerboat driving ‡ Golf (power cart) Canoeing (4 km or 2½ miles/hr) Horseback riding (walk) Playing piano and many musical instruments
3–4 METs 11–14 ml O_2/min/kg 4–5 kcal/min (70 kg person)	Brick laying, plastering Wheelbarrow (45.4 kg or 100 lb load) Machine assembly Trailer-truck in traffic Welding (moderate load) Cleaning windows	Walking (4.8 km or 3 miles/hr) Cycling (9.7 km or 6 miles/hr) Horseshoe pitching Volleyball (6-man noncompetitive) Golf (pulling bag cart) Archery Sailing (handling small boat) Fly fishing (standing with waders) Horseback (sitting to trot) Badminton (social doubles) Pushing light power mower Energetic musician
4–5 METs 14–18 ml O_2/min/kg 5–6 kcal/min (70 kg person)	Painting, masonry Paperhanging Light carpentry	Walking (5.6 km or 3½ miles/hr) Cycling (12.9 km or 8 miles/hr) Table tennis Golf (carrying clubs) Dancing (foxtrot) Badminton (singles) Tennis (doubles) Raking leaves Hoeing Many calisthenics
5–6 METs 18–21 ml O_2/min/kg 6–7 kcal/min (70 kg person)	Digging garden Shoveling light earth	Walking (6.4 km or 4 miles/hr) Cycling (16.1 km or 10 miles/hr) Canoeing (6.4 km or 4 miles/hr) Horseback ("posting" to trot) Stream fishing (walking in light current in waders) Ice or roller skating (14.5 km or 9 miles/hr)

CHART CONT. NEXT PAGE

6–7 METs 21–25 ml O_2/min/kg 7–8 kcal/min (70 kg person)	Shoveling 10/min (4.5 kg or 10 lbs)	Walking (8.0 km or 5 miles/hr) Cycling (17.7 km or 11 miles/hr) Badminton (competitive) Tennis (singles) Splitting wood Snow shoveling Hand lawn-mowing Folk (square) dancing Light downhill skiing Ski touring (4.0 km or 2½ miles/hr) (loose snow) Water skiing
7–8 METs 25–28 ml O_2/min/kg 8–10 kcal/min (70 kg person)	Digging ditches Carrying 36.3 kg or 80 lbs Sawing hardwood	Jogging (8.0 km or 5 miles/hr) Cycling (19.3 km or 12 miles/hr) Horseback (gallop) Vigorous downhill skiing Basketball Mountain climbing Ice hockey Canoeing *8.0 km or 5 miles/hr) Touch football Paddleball
8–9 METs 28–32 ml O_2/min/kg 10–11 kcal/min (70 kg person)	Shoveling 10/min (6.4 kg or 14 lbs)	Running (8.9 km or 5½ miles/hr) Cycling (20.9 km or 13 miles/hr) Ski touring /6.4 km or 4 miles/hr) (loose snow) Squash racquets (social) Handball (social) Fencing Basketball (vigorous)

10 plus METs
32 plus ml O_2/min/kg
11 plus kcal/min
(70 kg person)
	Shoveling 10/min
	(7.3 kg or 16 lbs)
		Running: 6 mph = 10 METs
		     7 mph = 11½ METs
		     8 mph = 13½ METs
		     9 mph = 15 METs
		     10 mph = 17 METs
		Ski touring (8 + km or 5+ miles/hr) (loose snow)
		Handball (competitive)
		Squash (competitive)

Reprinted from Fox SM, Naughton JP and Gorman PA: Physical Activity and Cardiovascular Health.

III. The exercise prescription; frequency and type of activity *Mod Concepts Cardiovasc Dis* 41:6. June 1972.

*includes resting metabolic needs.

† MET is the energy expenditure at rest, equivalent to approximately 3.5 ml O_2/kg body weight/minute.

‡ A major excess metabolic increase may occur due to excitement anxiety or impatience in some of these activities and a physician must assess his patient's psychological reactivity.

At 3 - 4 mets we learn that driving a trailer-truck in traffic is comparable to cleaning windows, which is comparable to pulling a golf cart or being an energetic musician. The chart is valuable in that it puts into perspective energy expenditure and calorie-use for various activities in daily life, and comparable activities in recreational pursuits. As you get farther down the chart, you begin to see the value of running, where a great number of calories can be burned and the aerobic base strengthened in a short time.

Here are some pointers for using the Air-Dyne: Adjust the seat so that your knee is slightly bent when one leg is extended and the corresponding pedal is at its most downward position. Get comfortable on the seat. Wear comfortable clothing. Have some additional clothes handy; the Air-Dyne produces a wind that cools you, but you may not need to be cooled this particular day, at your beginning slow speed. Don't worry about setting the timer at this point, because we'll take a very casual ride to get to know the machine. Grasp the handles firmly, as though you were going to push a lawnmower, put your feet on the pedals, and begin to gently turn them. Your arms will pump forward and back with handles. You'll notice that if you want the pedals to move faster, you not only have to push *faster*, but *harder*. Your effort is gauged and recorded on a dial on the bottom of your instrument panel. Don't push the dial past .5 until you get comfortable with the machine's sequence of movements.

At .5, you'll become accustomed to it very quickly and easily; the effort is minimal. Pedal for two minutes at this effort and then, just to feel how the machine functions, pedal harder to push the dial up to 1.0. You will notice that you had to increase the speed of the pedaling and handle-pushing as well as the force. This resistance approximates the real world. Back off, let the machine come to rest, and get off and walk a little to loosen your legs. Get in the habit of doing some light stretching exercises (see Jean Couch's *Runner's World Yoga Book* or her *Runner's World Stretching Book*) after each workout.

Now let's set up a progressive program.

BIG GOLD PROGRAM ALPHA

The title of this section sounds like a college football program/promotion in 1997. But it's a starter's program for the Air-Dyne. This program is geared for those who are in reasonably good condition, that have been exercising aerobically for about six months,

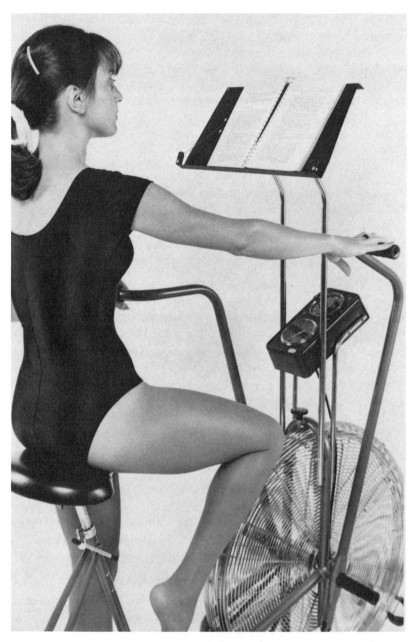

One of the clever options available is a reading stand, on which you can place this book while you exercise.

and that have had a physical if they're 30 or over. Even though I'd run more than a dozen marathons in the three years leading up to mounting "Big Gold," I approached it as I would any new exercise routine or regimen: with caution. If you're going through a change, say from no activity to activity, from swimming to bicycling, or from running to the Air-Dyne, you are going to begin using slightly different muscles and those muscles you've been using will be exercised in slightly different ways. By easing into the program you reduce the risk of sore muscles and injury. I would rather come away from the first few weeks on a new exercise routine feeling that I still had a lot left than hobble off looking for a hot bath and a doctor. You aren't going anywhere in such a hurry that you can't *ease* into new exercise programs.

Start by going short and gently. The first day you should not spend more than 15 minutes on the machine, and some of that time should go for a warmup and cooldown. Get aboard, set the timer, and start with five minutes at .5, five minutes at 1.0, and five minutes at .5. It may seem woefully inadequate, but if you had payed attention to your arms and legs during the workout, you'd have noticed that there were certain places on them where the effort was noticeable. If you had pushed it much farther than you did, the points of stress would have become even more noticeable, perhaps painful. I found it best to place the Air-Dyne workout into my routine after running a few miles. I would use it and then run a few miles more. By doing that, I noticed how the Air-Dyne worked other muscles. I would start training on the Air-Dyne and find very quickly that my muscles were being used in a slightly different way from running. I had to concentrate to keep the dial on the number I wanted, and that there was a definite physical effort involved. When I got off the machine my legs felt weak, as though I'd just done a track workout. When I began running again, I found my knee lift to be higher than it had been, but as a result of that unexpected sensation I had to back off on my pace because I found myself running awkwardly at first. Obviously, the Air-Dyne had stressed my leg muscles in slightly different directions with slightly different loads than they were used to with running. I felt that the Air-Dyne exercising would improve my running speed, because I had a similar sensation at track workouts after riding my bicycle regularly; the knee is lifted much higher in cycling than it is in running, and when you run after pedaling, the knee lift is more sure and more powerful.

When you begin on the Air-Dyne, you needn't abandon whatever other exercise you are doing, but attempt to work the Air-Dyne in with it. Using the Air-Dyne four times a week for 15 minutes a session, always followed with some stretching exercises, should be sufficient for the first few weeks. As you progress, you can build more strength by increasing the load you are using for those 15 minutes. For the first four weeks, then, the program would look like this:

Weeks 1 - 4
(15 minutes per session)

Day	Monday	Tuesday	Wednesday	Thursday	Friday	Saturday	Sunday
Week 1	.5/1/.5*	—	.5/1/.5	—	.5/1/.5	—	.5/1/.5
Week 2	.5/1/.5	—	.5/1/.5	—	.5/1/.5	—	.5/1/.5
Week 3	1/1.5/1	—	1/1.5/1	—	1/1.5/1	—	1/1.5/1
Week 4	1/1.5/1	—	1/1.5/1	—	1/1.5/1	—	1/1.5/1

*Each level should be held uniformly for 5 minutes, the lower levels serving as warm-up and cool-down periods.

The workouts on the Air-Dyne should be used either to supplement other exercising, or other exercising routines should be used to augment the Air-Dyne. The machine should not be used exclusively.

Progression for the subsequent weeks will not be as radical as they were for the first four weeks. Again, caution is the key word. You should be stressing your muscles, not straining them.

Weeks 5 - 10

Day	Monday	Tuesday	Wednesday	Thursday	Friday	Saturday	Sunday
Week 5	1/2/1	—	1/1.5/1	—	1/2/1	—	1/1.5/1
Week 6	1/2/1	—	1/1.5/1	—	1/2/1	—	1/1.5/1
Week 7	1/2/1	—	1/1.5/1	—	1/2/1	—	1/1.5/1
Week 8	1/2/1	—	1/2/1	—	1/2/1	—	1/2/1
Week 9	1/2.5/1	—	1/2/1	—	1/2.5/1	—	1/2/1
Week 10	1/2.5/1	—	1/2/1	—	1/2.5/1	—	1/2/1

From this point on, the workouts can be expanded and varied. Do not lock yourself into these workouts, however. If, at any time, you begin to feel sore or weak, back down to the workout of two weeks previous and stay there another week or two. The workouts outlined here are only suggestions, and are not carved in stone. It is always better to back off when you feel a potential for injury or excessive fatigue.

Once you have your first 10 weeks in, you can move up to occasional 20-minute workouts, perhaps starting at once a week. Your next five weeks would look like this:

Weeks 11 - 15

Day	Monday	Tuesday	Wednesday	Thursday	Friday	Saturday	Sunday
Week 11	1/2.5/1	—	1/2/2.5/1	—	1/2.5/1	—	1/2/1
Week 12	1/2.5/1	—	1/2/2.5/1	—	1/2.5/1	—	1/2/2/1
Week 13	1/2.5/1	—	1/2/2/1	—	1/2/2.5/1	—	1/2/1
Week 14	1/2/2/1	—	1/2.5/1	—	1/2/2.5/1	—	1/2/1
Week 15	1/2/2.5/1	—	1/2/1	—	1/2/2/1	—	1/2.5/1

What you are doing at this point is expanding approximately the energy necessary to stay healthy and fit according to Ken Cooper's guidelines. Much depends on your weight; as you'll recall the chart hinges on your body weight and is based on a 12-minute session on the Air-Dyne. But your workout in the 15th week is getting you close to being fit.

For many of you, though, merely being healthy and fit isn't enough. You want to be super-fit. For you enthusiastic folks, let's take the training program a bit farther.

Weeks 16 - 25

Day	Monday	Tuesday	Wednesday	Thursday	Friday	Saturday	Sunday
Week 16	1/2/3/2/1	—	1/2/2/1	—	1/2/3/3/1	—	1/2/2.5/1
Week 17	1/2/3/2/1	—	1/2/2.5/1	—	1/2/3/3/1	—	1/2/3/1
Week 18	1/2/3/3/1	—	1/2/2.5/1	—	1/3/2/3/1	—	1/2/3/1
Week 19	1/2/3/3/1	—	1/2/3.5/1	—	1/3/2/3/1	—	1/2.5/3/1
Week 20	1/2.5/3/2.5/1	—	1/2.5/3/1	—	1/2/3/3.5/1	—	1/2/3/1
Week 21	1/3/2.5/3/1	—	1/3/2/1	—	1/2/3.5/3/1	—	1/2/3/1
Week 22	1/3/3.5/3/1	—	1/2/3/1	—	1/2/3/4/1	—	1/3/2/1
Week 23	1/2/3/3.5/1	—	1/2/3/1	—	1/2/3/4/1	—	1/3/2/1
Week 24	1/2.5/4.5/1	—	1/2/2.5/1	—	1/2/4/3/1	—	1/2/3/1
Week 25	1/3/5/1	—	1/2/3/1	—	1/2/3/4/1	—	1/3/3/1

From this point on, by gauging your progress and your recovery time, you can program your own sessions on the Air-Dyne. Be careful, however, when you move forward into either more time slots or more effort. Each move forward should be followed by a recovery week, or longer. The body builds up endurance by stress and recovery. It is essential that you listen to your body, because it has ways of telling you when you have put it through enough. Train, don't strain.

Rest is important; it allows your body to heal the damage produced by stress and makes your body stronger for the next effort. In the previous schedules there are four days of work and three days of rest. In all except the first and last day of the week, there is a rest day between the work days. In the work days, there is a hard work day, but the next work day is relatively easier, so there are actually two hard/easy cycles involved in each week. All of the workouts from week 16 through week 25 are 20-25 minutes. You should not need much more than 25 minutes on the Air-Dyne. When you extrapolate beyond the 25th week, it is still advisable to keep the workouts in the 20-25 minute range, occasionally throwing in a 15-minute workout after a day that puts you at a higher training level.

Through all of it, though, pay attention to your body. If getting on the Air-Dyne is a real chore following a hard session two days before, modify your workout to allow yourself a break. Drop your recovery workout for that day from a 1/2/3/1 down to a 1/2.5/1 or a 1/2/1. If you feel really wiped out, just do five minutes at 1.5, enough to keep your legs loose. But don't baby yourself. Discipline is needed to pursue an ambitious exercise program, and it is often good for your body, mind and soul to push yourself through a workout on a day when you feel stale and listless for lack of inertia rather than because of physical fatigue. You should perk up considerably after the workout. If you don't, you probably do need rest.

Back off for physical problems. If you are doing a hard workout and you notice a twinge beginning in the outside of your knee, immediately back down on the effort, take a hot shower and forget the rest of the training session. The body almost always gives some preliminary indication that a part of it is receiving excessive strain. It may come in the guise of twinges and sore spots that persist from one workout to the next. Injury can also occur when you don't do your workouts smoothly and efficiently. For example, you may get sloppy and begin pushing the pedals from the sides instead of from directly overhead. You will probably put too much stress on the outside of your legs, ankles and feet, which can result in injury.

Assuming that your basic workouts are going along well, it is time to play some games with the machine. Let's set up some indoor running courses and workouts that you can throw in to your program once or twice a week. We'll break them down like this: LSD, fartlek, repetitions, road race and marathon.

GETTING HIGH ON LSD

The term "LSD" came into prominence during the 1960s with two groups of people: college students experimenting with drugs, and runners. In some instances, a person could be one and the same, an experimenter with drugs on campus and a runner. But the incidence of cross-over was limited. Runners were getting their own kind of "high" from their running and didn't necessarily need drugs.

The "LSD" of which I speak refers to "Long, Slow Distance." It was a training method that would revolutionize the world of running, and that would ultimately change the face of participant sports in America. It was largely responsible for the large number of seemingly normal Americans who took to running in a big way and who significantly altered their lifestyles to make room for running and exercise in their lives. It has essentially made long-distance running accessible to the masses, instead of allowing it to be hoarded by the elite runners of the world.

LSD is grounded in the theories of aerobic exercise. By running at a slow, comfortable pace, you can gradually increase your endurance until you can cover a lot of mileage. With LSD, more begets more. The more you run the longer you are able to run. The secret is to stay as comfortable as you can while you are running. A good sign of whether you are running comfortably is being able to hold a conversation while you run.

The benefits of LSD training are numerous. Your cardiorespiratory system is improved, your muscles toned, your chance of injury is much less than with hard training (as long as you are smooth and fluid in your stride, and you use the correct footwear), and you gain self-esteem from covering distance that a year before seemed long even in an automobile.

The same type of training can be applied to your Air-Dyne. Once in shape and on agreeable terms with the machine, you will find a setting where you reach maximum efficiency. It may be at a point between 2 and 2.5 or it may be higher. Just as in bicycling you should find the right, cadence where you are most efficient; you can pump for hours at that cadence. Each of you has a point of perfect rhythm within your bodies.

As your condition improves, your cadence will likely increase, too. Once you have found the ideal cadence try to hold it for a sustained exercise period.

As with the progressive workouts on the Air-Dyne, a warmup is very important. Five minutes at an effort of 1 will be sufficient to warm the muscles for an LSD effort. The jump from 1 to your efficient cadence should come smoothly and effortlessly. If it is 2.5, move up to 2.5 cleanly and without any undue effort, even if it takes a full minute to get from 1 to 2.5. Maintain regular breathing. As in running, you should be able to talk while you are exercising, otherwise you're training too hard for an LSD workout.

If you are already doing 25-minute workouts, move your first LSD workout up to 30 minutes, using the first five as warmup and the last five as a cooldown. Do not push too hard on your first sessions. Increases should be done logically, smoothly, and in small increments. You may take four weeks or longer of LSD before moving from 30 minutes up to 35. The LSD will be much easier, too, if it is alternated with the various-paced workouts. Don't just stay in LSD all the time, or you'll quickly settle your body into a top end of whatever your efficient cadence is. Of course, such excursions into regions above your cadence have their own classifications, if you happen to be doing them in the middle of your LSD workouts.

A SMORGASBORD OF FARTLEK

The term "fartlek" comes from the Swedes and means "speed play." The Swedes like to think that they invented speed play, but our childhoods are filled with play that resembles fartlek in design. If you've ever watched a child run, it is always erratic, and seldom, if ever, even-paced. Children are like hummingbirds, sprinting about, pausing for a moment here or there when some bright object on the ground catches their attention, and then flitting off again at top speed. In a crude and primitive way, this constitutes fartlek's principles.

Fartlek is a fun way of simulating boring track workouts. Their results are much the same, however. They can be done on the roads or, as the Swedes like to do them, along forest trails. Your pace is usually dictated by hills, so there is no chance of dropping into a set pace and staying there for a half-hour. The essence of fartlek follows: a warm up of a few minutes; speed pacing, in which you pick out a point farther ahead on the trail you are running, and increase your pace until you reach that object, whether it be a boulder or a telephone pole; then you back down again for a period after you've reached that goal, so that your body can recover from the increased exertion. The entire run, then, is built around a smooth, even pace that is periodically interrupted by surges. Fartlek on the roads is usually done by using telephone poles as markers. The runner surges between two telephone poles, and then backs down to an easy pace for the next pole, and so on.

In applying fartlek to your Air-Dyne or an exercise bicycle, you will use the concept differently. Using the LSD cadence as your base line for the workout, you will increase the tempo at random. If you have found that your ideal cadence is at 2.5, push yourself up to 3.5 for a minute and then drop back to 2.5 for two minutes of recovery, then take a 30-second surge to 4.5, dropping back for about 1½ minutes of recovery at 2.5. Remember to give yourself a one-minute warmup at 1, and a cooldown at 1. Use your second minute getting reacquainted with your 2.5 cadence before making a surge.

Don't make a fartlek workout as long as your longest LSD workout, because the extra effort of surging takes a lot out of you. As a general rule, hold your first fartlek efforts to at least 10 minutes less than your longest LSD ride. Be sure, when using the Air-Dyne, to let your arms do some of the work. Fartlek running makes exaggerated use of the arms when going up hills and initiating surges. Perhaps, if you are in need of goals and find it easier to stick to a set schedule, you can make up your workouts before you ever mount the Air-Dyne. If you're doing 30-minute LSD workouts at a cadence level of 2.5, you might want to work up a fartlek workout like this:

>   60 seconds — 1
>   60 seconds — 2.5
>   30 seconds — 3.5
>   15 seconds — 5
>   60 seconds — 2.5
>   90 seconds — 3.5
>   60 seconds — 2.5
>   30 seconds — 4
>   30 seconds — 2.5
>   60 seconds — 4
>   60 seconds — 2.5
>   120 seconds — 3.5
>   60 seconds — 2.5

30 seconds — 5.5
90 seconds — 2.5
90 seconds — 4
30 seconds — 2.5
15 seconds — 7
90 seconds — 2.5
60 seconds — 1

The workout is 20 minutes long and features plenty of varied peaks, with heavy stress (level 7) kept to a minimum and saved for the end. A series of progressively more difficult peaks lead up to it. Don't put the maximum stress too early in the workout. Make sure that you spend one minute, preferably two or three, at the 1 setting to give your legs a cooldown as a final effort. Prep yourself for the fartlek workout by going easy on the previous workout and also take it easy during the subsequent training day. When you come to a stop, get off the machine and walk around a bit—for as much as 15 minutes to keep the tightness out of your legs. Then, do some stretching exercises while your muscles are still warm.

You might not like the seemingly random approach to training that characterizes fartlek. You might want to be more regular and more precise with your workouts. The answer for you is "interval" or "track" workouts.

THE REGULARITY OF REPETITIONS

Most new runners or those who run strictly in road races despise the track. It is like a dungeon to them, a place where they feel trapped. On the roads they see themselves running free, roaming where they will. The track, however, provides a precisely measured distance, on which the runner can practice pace and work toward increasing speed potential. For someone who has spent virtually every training mile on the roads, a shift in mental gears is required for doing track workouts. The track is an enclosed arena where there is no fear of being run over by cars, there are no unexpected potholes that will sneak up on you, and you can work with measured distances instead of those estimated on the road.

There is no place better for a road racer to sharpen his skills than on the track. Most world-class road racers use the track when they are working to peak for a big race; they seldom use it more than twice a week, though.

For the home exerciser who craves the precise, the mechanical, the predictable, the perfectly regular and regulated, a repetitions program can be an excellent method of pushing back the aerobic threshold.

Such a program is also easy to set up on the Air-Dyne as long as you follow the same principles of track we've been discussing: 1) Always take a warmup and a cooldown. 2) Increase your effort gradually at a pace you can adapt to easily. 3) Keep your time on hard workouts (which fartlek and repetitions are) to about 67 percent or less of your LSD workouts.

To show how easy a repetition program is to set up, let's put one together.

60 seconds – 1
60 seconds – 1.5
30 seconds – 2.5
60 seconds – 1.5
30 seconds – 2.5
60 seconds – 1.5
30 seconds – 2.5
60 seconds – 1.5
30 seconds – 2.5
60 seconds – 1.5
30 seconds – 2.5
60 seconds – 1.5
30 seconds – 2.5
60 seconds – 1.5
30 seconds – 2.5
60 seconds – 1.5
60 seconds – 1

If you think that such a workout would be bad-mouthed by people who prefer fartlek, you are correct. But all repetition workouts do not have to be precisely the same. Many runners use a pyramid rep workout, which you can easily incorporate into an Air-Dyne program. The pyramid principle is to make each effort a bit harder (or longer) until you reach the maximum goal for that day, and then to turn around and come back down the ladder. The following program would be an example:

60 seconds – 1
60 seconds – 1.5

30 seconds – 2
60 seconds – 1.5
30 seconds – 2.5
60 seconds – 1.5
30 seconds – 3
60 seconds – 1.5
30 seconds – 3.5
60 seconds – 1.5
30 seconds – 4
60 seconds – 1.5
30 seconds – 4.5
60 seconds – 1.5
30 seconds – 5
60 seconds – 1.5
30 seconds – 5.5
60 seconds – 1.5
30 seconds – 5
60 seconds – 1.5
30 seconds – 4.5
60 seconds – 1.5
30 seconds – 4
60 seconds – 1.5
30 seconds – 3.5
60 seconds – 1.5
30 seconds – 3
60 seconds – 1.5
30 seconds – 2.5
60 seconds – 1.5
30 seconds – 2
60 seconds – 1.5
60 seconds – 1

Now that's quite an ambitious workout and one that should hold your muscles in spasm for about two days. It's 25½ minutes long, and shouldn't be done unless you are already comfortably and regularly doing about 40-minute LSD workouts. The pattern calls for an increase of .5 each time you complete a 60-second recovery at 1.5, until you hit the maximum of 5.5, and then you gradually return to your starting point, coming down .5 each time.

Some repetition workouts, of course, go through sets of hard efforts at various distances, and that can be approximated on the

Air-Dyne, too. Suppose, for instance, that at the track you were doing six 110-yard wind sprints with a 110-yard jog between, followed by four 220-yard sprints with a 220-yard jog between, finishing with two 440-yard hard efforts, with a 440-yard jog between. Don't forget the mile warmup and the mile cooldown. You could come up with a program something like this:

     60 seconds – 1
     60 seconds – 1.5
     15 seconds – 5.5
     45 seconds – 1.5
     15 seconds – 5.5
     45 seconds – 1.5
     15 seconds – 5.5
     45 seconds – 1.5
     15 seconds – 5.5
     45 seconds – 1.5
     15 seconds – 5.5
     45 seconds – 1.5
     15 seconds – 5.5
     45 seconds – 1.5
     30 seconds – 5
     60 seconds – 1.5
     30 seconds – 5
     60 seconds – 1.5
     30 seconds – 5
     60 seconds – 1.5
     30 seconds – 5
     60 seconds – 1.5
     60 seconds – 4
     90 seconds – 1.5
     60 seconds – 4
     90 seconds – 1.5
     60 seconds – 1

The number of variations you can come up with is limited only by your own imagination, inclination and inventiveness. And by your physical capacities at the time. There is no reason to rush yourself into a maximum workout without the proper groundwork. Remember that you should always use the hard/easy method in your training/exercise programs. Your next scheduled workout following a repetition session should be LSD.

Some people will find their optimum levels set for them because of time restraints in their daily lives. Others, however, will continue to explore their bodies, gradually progressing, over a period of months and years, to hour-long sessions on the Air-Dyne. That is not so hard to imagine, because an option with the unit is a reading stand that allows you to read the newspaper or a book while putting in your hour's worth of LSD work each session. Or you can watch television. When you get comfortable doing long distances, there is only one thing left to try: a marathon.

MARATHON MADNESS

Many people who run marathons should not be doing so. Many of them run marathons because it seems the thing to do, because other people are doing them, because by doing them, they have something to talk about at cocktail parties. Or it may be the chance to thrust that middle finger in front of the nose of passing time, saying, in effect, "See there, I may be getting older, but if I can run 26 miles, 385 yards, I'm not as old as you led me to believe!"

It always astounds me to see people start running casually, and within a matter of a month, start talking about running a marathon—despite the fact that they had never run a race in their lives! They then embark on a full-fledged running program, enter a marathon, suffer and toil mightily through it in five or six hours, and consequently drop out of running entirely. Crazy!

For many others, however, the marathon is the next logical step in their competitive ladders. They run easy miles, then 10Ks, 20Ks and half-marathons and eventually want to challenge the marathon distance. They train wisely, relying on the experience they have gained from all their training and many races. They usually run a satisfying marathon.

The same positive approach can be taken with the exercise cycle. Although the effort required to keep the cycle going for a long time seems formidable at first, it is just a matter of sticking with it until you find yourself becoming stronger and aerobically fit.

It is certainly a challenge to gradually increase the length of your workout. Fighting off boredom isn't a problem if you're prepared. Clamping a pair of stereo headphones on your head so that you can listen to your favorite music while pumping yourself blue in the face is a pleasant way of burning up calories and building muscle strength and tone. Or watching TV or reading a book. Or just let your mind drift as your body finds its ideal pace and settles down for a long workout.

It is not wrong to devise a challenge toward which you can aim all of your training, and a marathon-like effort on the Air-Dyne isn't inconceivable. But you should contemplate such an event with care. A great deal of preparation must go into the marathon. You will, of course, have certain advantages over running outdoors in your effort:

1) Ideal environment—You can regulate your environment to what suits you. You won't get rained or snowed on, and you won't get sunburned.

2) Easy support—You can have one of your family or a friend standing by with a supply of fluids and ade or, if you want to do a solo effort, you can place a table next to your exercise cycle, with all the fluids and support materials you might need during your effort.

3) Flexible starting time—Since it is your marathon, you are the race director and can set your own starting time.

4) Convenience—You can essentially "create" your marathon for your Air-Dyne by putting together a program that will approximate that maximum sustained effort; in other words, your marathon can be accomplished by a combination of time/effort that is logical and customized to your state of training. It does not have to work out to exactly 26 miles, 385 yards, although the Air-Dyne does feature an odometer that can be used in that way. Your "marathon" would be an effort greater (longer and more sustained) than your previous best effort by perhaps a factor of 25 percent. We will discuss that shortly.

5) Comforts—Since the "race" is being conducted in the comfort of your own home, and will be stationary, you can employ all of the previously mentioned options that indoor exercise provides or you can tough it out by putting the bike in a lonely room, and concentrate on the "race" as though it were a real one.

These advantages make the effort more convenient than a marathon on the roads, but no amount of accessories or assistance is going to belittle the actual effort required to accept the challenge and match it.

So how should you go about setting it up?

There are several ways of doing it.

1) Straight distance. The Air-Dyne (and most other exercise cycles) features an odometer, and you could simply mount the cycle and pump away until the odometer has put 26.2 miles on it. Unfortunately, that isn't very accurate. A mile ridden on a bicycle isn't as demanding as a mile of running. So, if you want to do a marathon on an exercise cycle, you would have to use a setting that approximates level ground (unless you want to make it a hilly marathon course) and pump away until the odometer reached 104.8 miles. The idea would be to keep as steady a pace as possible, with the resistance set at level ground—unless you felt particularly strong, in which case you could adjust the setting for effort that would approximate a course with some hills.

2) Resistance distance. By increasing the resistance you must go up against, you can logically put out a marathon effort by covering less distance. This becomes a mathematical nightmare, however, as you calculate how much more effort equals how much less distance. The two are not directly proportional.

3) Effort-adjusted distance. This method relies on your previous best efforts on the Air-Dyne, in which you figure out the pace you have been working at, adjusting a target "time" at that effort that translates to 26.2 miles. Again, this is a mathematical nightmare. But it can be done.

4) Approximate effort/time. This is perhaps the easiest way, and although it is not as precise as other methods, it can be fun and comes close to producing the required effort. Here's how it works:

> 4 hours at an effort of "1"
> 3½ hours at an effort of "2"
> 3 hours at an effort of "3"
> 2½ hours at an effort of "4"

Using the latter method of doing your "marathon" is, admittedly, a sort of haphazard way of doing it, but it reflects what I feel should be inherent in anything as left-of-center as an Air-Dyne Marathon: that you do it seriously, but with a lighthearted attitude. If you pump away for three hours at an effort of "3" you can be sure that you have put out effort comparable to running a three-hour marathon.

TWO REVOLUTIONS BEYOND

In June of 1979 I ran a 24-hour track race. It was a charity affair. During the race, held at Huntington Beach, California, ultra-marathon superman Park Barner of Pennsylvania set a world record, covering more than 160 miles. It was later disallowed because the scoring was not done exactly according to the rules laid down by the sanctioning body that oversees such silly events. But nonetheless it was thrilling watching Park perform; his effort was supreme and profound. A soft-spoken, bashful guy with a precise wit, Park is far from what one pictures as being macho. He doesn't run for that ego need.

He and those who do the same madness on the track are very rare critters, competing in an arena that is still very much uncrowded. I mention them merely because someone who decides to do a "marathon" on an Air-Dyne is likely to be lying in a tub of hot water afterward wondering, "What can I do to top that?"

Well, the imagination—although it boggles—can conceive things beyond the famed Air-Dyne Marathon. I'm not sure it has to be pushed beyond the "marathon" point, though. Why contemplate locking yourself in your rec room to pedal away for 24 hours? What the purpose? Doing a "marathon" goes well beyond mere fitness anyway, right?

Enough is enough, right?

Right.

Did I mention another of my heroes? Don Choi. He revived the six-day races during 1980 after they'd been dead and buried for many, many decades. Right. Six days on the track. Running around and around and around, traveling hundreds of miles and staying all that time in the same place. You could take a week's vacation, get teams of friends to come by to help you by feeding you drinks and easily-digestible foods, and you could pedal your Air-Dyne for six days.

Or, you could forget that nonsense and stick to your basic fitness, doing a 10K run on your Air-Dyne every once in a while to burn off the extra competitive juices that bubble up.

Your body will thank you for ignoring this final section on exercise cycles. And your Air-Dyne will thank you for *not* putting it through 24 hours of non-stop use.

But it does make you wonder what Park Barner or Don Choi could do on an Air-Dyne . . .

5

Floor Games
by Rhonda Provost

Muscle contraction is a very complicated process. It involves a great number of sequential and simultaneous events that are caused by the mechanical, chemical and electrical systems of the body. The exploration of such intricate relationships and coordination of systems, except to know that they happen with every movement we make, lies outside the scope of this book. But I will explain certain "muscle mechanisms." Knowledge of such processes will assist you in achieving a maximum state of fitness. Once you understand what is involved in muscle activity you will tend to be more patient with your body. After all, strenuous exercise is almost always a voluntary experience.

We learned in Chapter 3 that neither bones nor muscles alone can hold the body upright. Bones are too irregularly shaped to balance one upon the other, so the only way your body can remain erect is for your muscles to pull the bones in opposition to gravity, which is pulling on your body at all times. Muscles exert this pull against gravity by virtue of their property of tonicity.

Tonus is a state of steady, partial contraction that occurs as a result of continuous nerve impulses coming to the muscle from the spinal cord. The amount of tone you have varies, but is present at all times in healthy muscle. Your muscles, particularly the ones that help you stand erect, are so arranged in your body that they gently stretch over your joints. When you stretch your muscles you trigger messages that cause their contraction. You can and should take advantage of tonicity by exercising on a regular basis, because muscle tends to contract more forcibly after it is slightly stretched. Thus, stretching contributes greatly to increased muscle tone.

Muscle, like all body tissue, is composed of cells. For any cell in the body to perform the functions for which it is designed, energy is required. This energy comes from within the cell itself; for any sustained level of activity, such as the type discussed in this chapter, additional oxygen is necessary for the production of enough energy to enable the muscles to continue their performance for a long time. The consumption of this energy results in the formation of waste products, which then need to be eliminated from the body.

Regular, forceful muscular activity causes the muscle to enlarge with time, allowing more room for additional oxygen to be transported. With the muscle's actual increase in power comes a concommitant increase in its ability to maintain this power by providing larger muscle fibers and more space for the metabolic processes to take place. (Do not worry, ladies. Females do not possess enough of the hormone testosterone necessary to achieve the well-developed musculature you see in men. So you can exercise as long as you want without looking like the female version of The Incredible Hulk.)

Although many systems are called into play during exercise, the most important is the cardiovascular system; without its continuous action of pumping blood, the needs of the exercising body cannot be met. One of the many functions that muscles serve, by virtue of their tone, is to aid in the return of blood to the heart. That's because highly toned muscles lend support to the vessels that help transport blood to and from the heart. This effect is significantly enhanced during exercise, when the muscles are providing a massage-like effect on the walls of these vessels. The resulting increased blood flow to the heart means improved blood supply leaving the heart and an increased ability for your body to provide the necessary oxygen and nutrients to the active muscle, as well as thr removal of waste products. The final result is increased muscle efficiency—muscles performing an equal or greater amount of work at less energy cost.

When a muscle is engaged in an activity that causes prolonged, repetitious contractions, it progressively loses its initial forcefulness of contraction and the ability to meet its metabolic needs. Consequently, the muscle fails to supply the same power after a given time. Muscle fatigue ensues.

Although functions regulating muscle contractions are still operating, the available energy stores within the muscle itself become depleted. Lactic acid, which is an end-product of metabolism, also contributes to this fatigue because it fails to be adequately eliminated. Muscle strength and the elimination of waste products, causing sore, stiff muscles diminishes. For the unconditioned, these symptoms are commonplace. Do not be discouraged should you find yourself fatigued and weak halfway through these routines. Indeed, anticipate it. Be patient. Give your body a chance. With time, it will accept and accommodate. Prolonged muscle activity does lead to increased muscle endurnace.

Because prolonged muscle activity depletes available energy stores, a workout that is *too* vigorous for *too* long a time will not be beneficial. Your muscles will not, and in fact are incapable of, responding as well. The chance for injury is also increased, so although these exercises may take longer, all the routines are not to be done as vigorously. Stretching and position-holding is spaced so that you can take a break in a vigorous oxygen-consuming workout, but continue moving so that you remain "warmed up." These guidelines should enable you to enjoy this series of exercises to its fullest. Some exercises do not have specific time frames listed. Because with time and experience you will enjoy assuming and maintaining some of the positions, the amount of time you spend on each exercise should be up to you.

I. The Rockettes' Revival—Stand with your feet together and your arms out to your sides, parallel to the floor. Begin by raising your right leg, bending it at the knee. Hold it out in front of you like a Rockette at Radio City Music Hall. Maintain this position for the count of 20. Proceed to straighten your leg, kicking it up and out to the front of you. Return it, without letting it touch the floor. Now raise it while straightened, up and out to the side of you, again for a count of 20. Drop it again to the starting position without letting it touch the floor and immediately raise it in a straightened position up and out in back of you, holding to a 20 count. Repeat this sequence 10 times, balancing yourself on your left leg. Now, switch and do the same to the right leg.

II. The Back-Under Reach—Stand with your legs spread about two feet and place your hands on your hips. Now bend at the hips until the upper portion of your body is parallel to the floor. Keep your back straight. Stretch your arms out in front of you in a swimming dive and bounce toward the floor eight times. Now,

The Rockettes' Revival

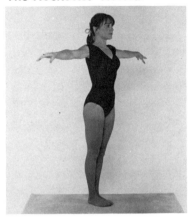
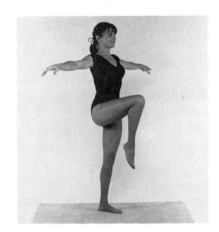
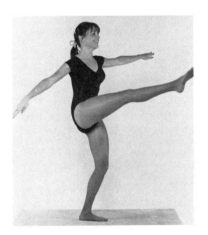

Assume a standing position, with arms out to sides, parallel to the floor. Raise the right leg, bending it at the knee. Hold it for a 20 count, and then kick it out in front of you, bringing it back and sending it out to the side. Finish the sequence by balancing yourself on your left leg and holding your leg out behind you. Now repeat the sequence 10 times before doing the entire sequence over with the other leg.

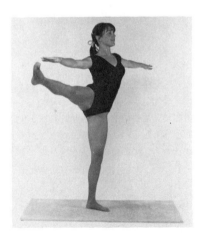
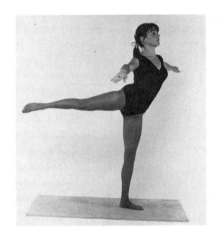

place the palms of your hands flat in front of you on the floor and bounce eight times. Clasp your hands and with arms outstretched, aim down between your legs, stretching your arms behind you toward the floor; bounce toward the back eight times. With outstretched arms, return to a position parallel to the floor and bounce eight times, then resume standing with hands on hips to an eight count. Repeat the sequence five times.

III. Ballet Bends—Using a ballet bar, kitchen counter, or some stable object that is at least waist-high or higher, stand with your left side arm's length away. With your feet together, hold the bar with your left hand and keep your right hand out to the side, parallel to the floor. Hold your tummy in and keep your back straight; shift your pelvis left toward the bar and simultaneously drop your right hand to your right knee. With pelvis tilted and and leaning into the bar, bounce 10 times. Now, reverse the tilt of the pelvis to the right while leaning into it and bring your right hand over your head in a circular fashion, stretching as far as you can. Again, bounce 10 times. Repeat this entire sequence five times. Turn and do it from the other side. You will feel a stretch in your waist and the outer thigh.

The Back-Under Reach

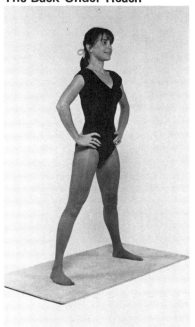

Stand with your legs spread and your hands on your hips.

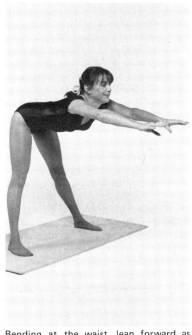

Bending at the waist, lean forward as though getting ready to dive.

cont'd next page

The Back-Under Reach (cont'd)

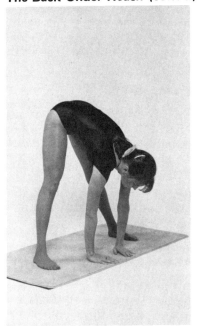

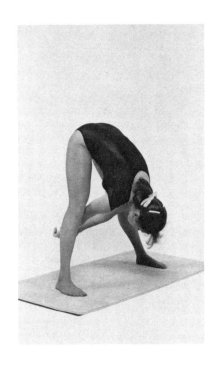

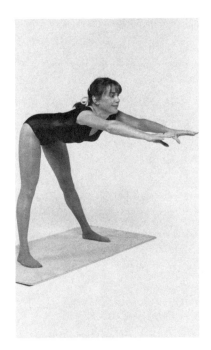

Now place the palms of your hands on the floor in front of you and bounce eight times. Then clasp your hands together and shoot them out behind you, going through your legs, bouncing eight times. Then come back to the dive position and bounce eight times before returning to the original position.

Ballet Bends

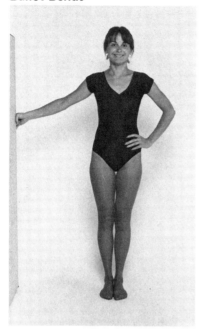

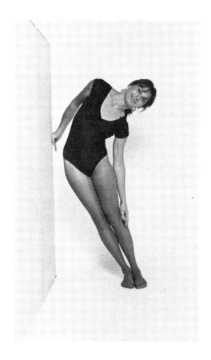

Stand at arm's length away from a solid object waist high or higher. Shift your pelvis toward the support object, dropping your outside hand to your knee. Bounce 10 times. Then reverse the tilt of the pelvis, bringing your hand up over your head in a circular fashion. Again bounce 10 times. Make the feeling of stretching as apparent as you can.

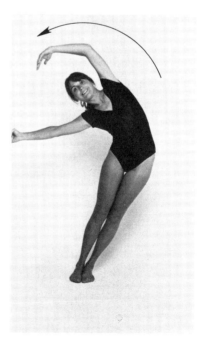

Toe Lifts

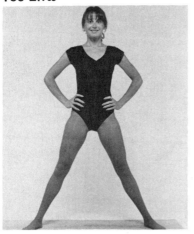
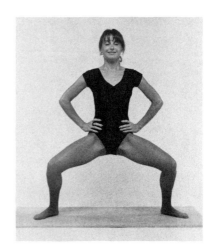
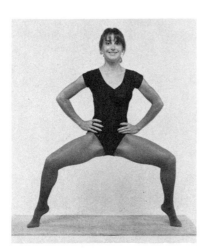

This one is a great strength-builder for the legs. Start with your legs spread about two feet, and go into a squat, using only the legs throughout the entire exercise. Raise yourself on your toes, and then straighten your legs besides. Then lower yourself off your toes to your starting position, and repeat.

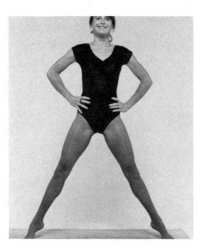
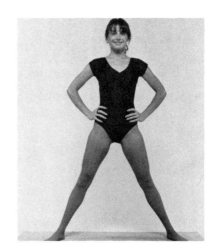

IV. Toe Lifts—Stand straight with your hands on your hips and your legs apart about two feet. Now squat. Lift your heels off the floor while your toes remain planted and while you are still squatting. Now stand up while still lifting your heels and rest the feet flat on the floor once you are standing. Repeat this eight times. When you come up for the eighth time, continue to lift the heels while standing straight with your hands on your hips. Now, lift yourself on your toes and squat (while still on your toes). Flatten your feet while squatting and resume standing. Repeat this eight times. Repeat the entire sequence twice.

V. The Lunge & Thrust—This exercise is actually a series of combined, smaller exercises. It is meant, however, to be done as one exercise. To facilitate matters, I will subdivide the exercise into its components and label them "A" through "F."

A. Stand with your legs spread and feet facing the right side. Place your hands on your hips. Lunge to the right as though you were fencing, bending your right leg at the knee and keeping your left leg straight, and then return to the upright position. Repeat this eight times.

B. Lunge to the right, bending your right leg at the knee and keeping your left leg straight and try to place the palms of your hands on the floor on either side of your right foot. Drop your head to your right knee and proceed to raise and lower your buttocks by straightening and flexing your right leg. Keep your left leg as straight as possible. Do this eight times. After raising your buttocks on the eighth count, keep your left leg straight, hold your right ankle with both hands, and touch your nose to your right knee eight times.

C. Repeat exercise A.

D. In an upright position, with your legs still spread, face forward. Your feet should now be facing front also. Hold your arms out straight in front of you and drop so that you rest on your right leg, knee bent, and your left leg is out straight to your side resting on your left heel. In that position, bounce eight times. No hands! Finish by remaining in that position and shifting your body weight while squatting from your right to your left leg and back to your right again.

E. Repeat exercise A.

F. Still facing the right side, drop to your left knee. Now, grab your left ankle with your left hand and hold your right arm straight out in front of you. Lean forward on your right leg and pull your left heel to your buttock and hold to the count of eight. Now repeat the entire routine and work your left side.

The Lunge & Thrust

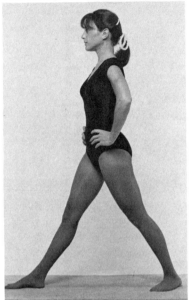

Stand with your feet apart, as though you'd been caught in the act of taking one giant step. Put your hands on your hips, because you want the work to come entirely from the legs during the initial movements. Now bend at the knee of the forward leg, keeping the trailing leg straight.

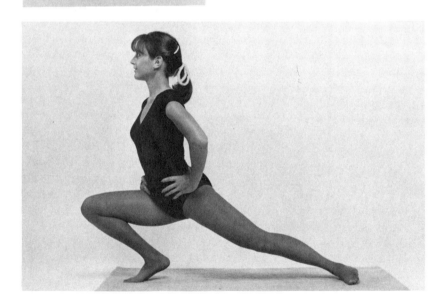

cont'd next page

The Lunge & Thrust (cont'd)

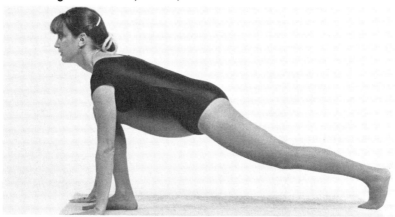

On your next lunge, try to place your palms flat on the floor, then raise buttocks.

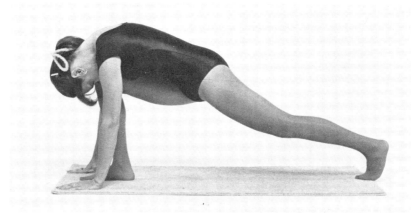

Now, lower the buttocks; raise and lower them a total of eight times.

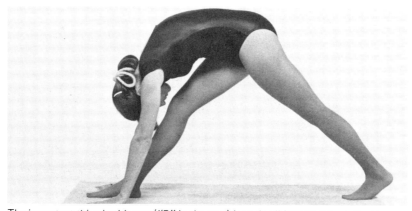

The important thing in this one ("B" in the text) is to do all bouncing from the hips.

cont'd next page

The Lunge & Thrust (cont'd)

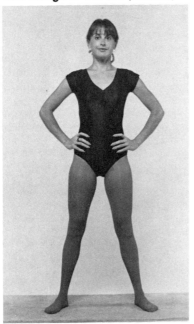

This is a relatively easy way of building leg strength and flexibility. (In the text, it is "D".) Start in a simple standing position with hands on hips. Then drop to support yourself on one leg, the other extended out to serve as a balance factor; keep your arms out in front of you so that all movements are made through the legs.

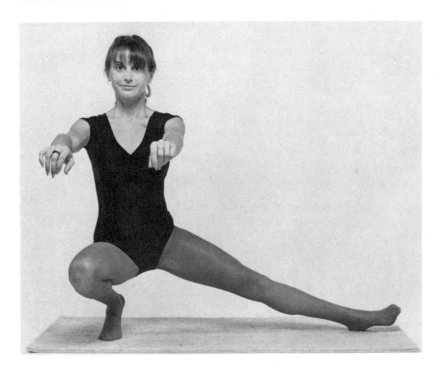

cont'd next page

The Lunge & Thrust (cont'd)

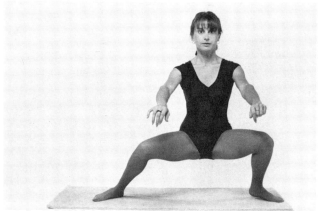

When you're done with one leg, shift yourself across to the other leg and work that one.

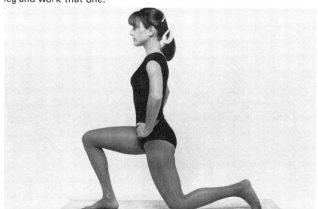

For section "F" in the sequence, drop to the left knee, with hands still on hips.

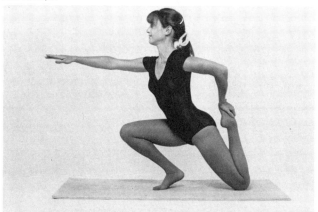

Now lean forward while grasping your trailing ankle and putting your leading arm out.

VI. Knee Drops—Sit on the floor with straight legs spread in front of you about two feet apart. While sitting straight with your tummy pulled in, place your hands behind your head with your fingers entwined. Now bend at your hips to touch your right elbow to your left knee, and return to the sitting position while continuing through to touch your left elbow to your right knee. Repeat this 30 times.

VII. The Long Sit-Up—Sit on the floor with your back straight and legs together straight in front of you. Now lie down with your arms outstretched above your head. Proceed to sit up and while sitting draw your knees to your chest and do not let your feet touch the floor. When you achieve a sitting position, your arms should be parallel to the floor on either side of each knee. Immediately return to the reclining position with your legs out straight and your arms above your head. Do 10 of these and without stopping proceed to a variation of this, as described here. Continue in essentially the same fashion, except, when in the sitting position alternate by having *both* arms on *either* side of each knee. Do a total of 20 of these. The total number of sit-ups for this exercise should be 30.

VIII. Split 'n' Sit—While lying on your back, lift and spread your legs above you. Hold them in this position while you do 20 sit-ups, touching the floor in front of you and between your legs with your outstretched hands.

IX. The Pretzel—Immediately after completing the sit-ups, raise your legs and pelvis straight above your head, supporting your pelvis with your hands while resting on the back of your upper arms. Concentrate on keeping your back straight and your legs perpendicular to the floor. Try to lower your straightened leg behind your head to the floor while keeping your left leg straight above you. Return your right leg up to your left leg straight above you. Proceed to drop your left leg behind your head to the floor while keeping your right leg straight above you. Repeat this entire sequence 20 times.

Now, simultaneously lower both straightened legs together until they are parallel to the floor at a point about six inches from the floor. Flex your toes toward the floor. Your arms should be down at your sides with your palms flat on the floor. Now hold this position to the count of 20.

Maintain this position while you spread your legs as far apart as you can. Continue to keep your legs straight and hold to a

Knee Drops

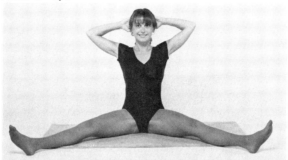

Spread your legs and keep your back straight and put your hands behind your head.

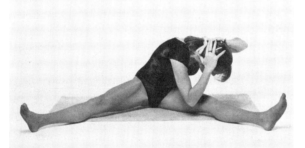

Now drop your right elbow to your left knee, doing all bending at the hips.

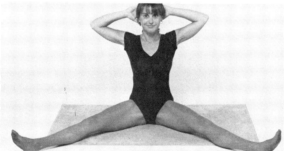

Come back up to the starting position, still keeping the back straight.

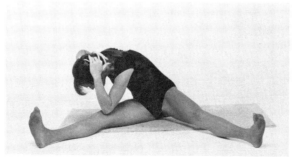

Now go down with your left elbow heading for your right knee cap. Repeat 30 times.

The Long Sit-Up

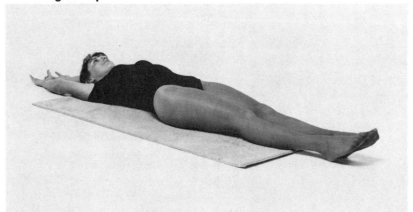

Pretend that you're Superman and that you're flying over tall buildings upside down.

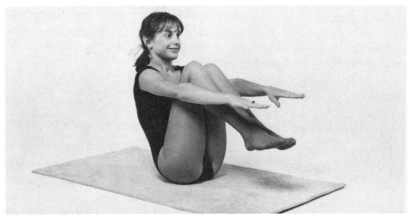

Now, very smoothly, come to a sitting position by bringing up arms and legs.

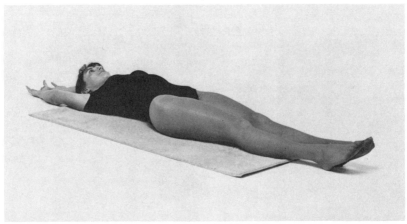

Then, return to the Superman flying position; do this 10 times.

cont'd next page

The Long Sit-Up (cont'd)

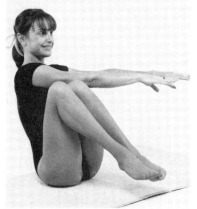

Now do the same sequence over, but when you come up, put the arms to the side.

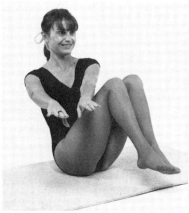

On every other sit-up, put your arms out to the opposite side.

Splt 'n' Sit

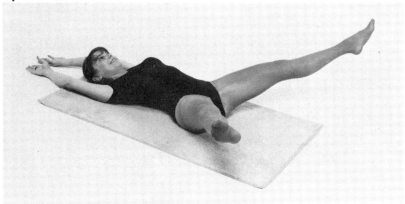

In the Superman flying position again, but with your legs spread and off the floor.

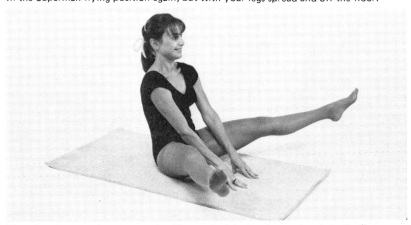

Then, keeping your legs there and rolling on the hip, touch your hands to the floor.

count of 20. Now drop your still straight legs and flexed feet to the floor. Hold for a count of 20. Now join your straightened legs together and hold for a count of 20.

Next raise your arms to lie straight on the floor above your head. Raise your straightened legs so that they again remain parallel to the floor with your feet flexed toward the floor. Hold for a count of 20. Again spread your legs as far as you can and hold for the count of 20. Now lower your legs to the floor and hold for a count of 20. Finally, join them, straightened, for the count of 20. Then drop your knees to either side of your head and hold for a count of 10. Return to a position flat on the floor.

The Pretzel

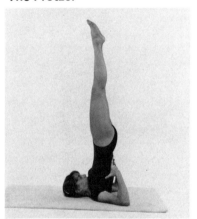
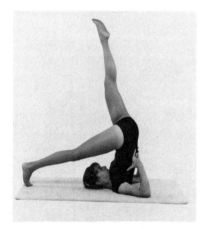
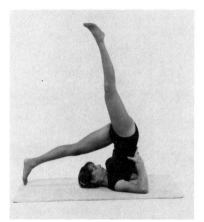
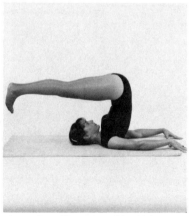

In this one, the pictures pretty much speak for themselves. Move smoothly, Make every motion controlled.

cont'd next page

The Pretzel (cont'd)

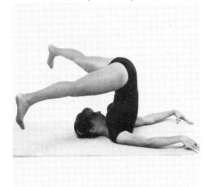
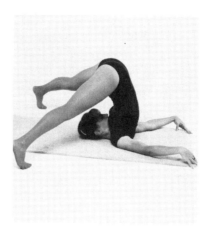
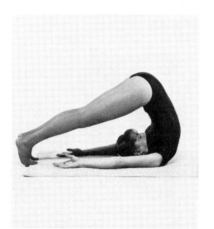
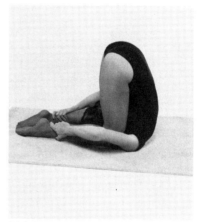

Don't despair if it doesn't come to you easily; Rich has been trying for a year to get his knees by his ears.

X. Nosey Knee—Lie on your back with your left leg straight, and place your left foot under a heavy chair or some similar object that will help you remain immobile for this stretch. Hold your straightened right leg perpendicular to the floor. Keep that left leg straight while you grasp the ankle of your straightened right leg. While keeping both legs straight, raise yourself enough to touch your nose to your right knee to the count of 20. Switch sides and repeat.

XI. Back Bend—In order to get the feel of this one (and to give your thighs, buttocks, back, and arms a workout at the same time), try it first while you lie on the floor. Draw your feet up as close as you can to your buttocks. Now plant the palms of your hands at the level of your shoulders. Begin by lifting your pelvis off the floor. Then, as you attempt to lift the upper part of your body you can assist yourself in that initial lift by rolling back on your occiput (the back of your head). Hold that position for as long as you want. Extend your head as far back as you can. Attempt to view the floor behind you. Return to the lying position and do it again.

XII. Straight Leg—Lie on your back with arms straight out at your sides and legs straight. Draw your knees together to your chest, extend them straight together directly above you and lower them slowly *almost* to the floor. Do 20 repetitions. Now raise yourself to your elbows and repeat 15 of the same cycles. Conclude by supporting yourself on your palms with your arms straight and performing 10 of the same sequence.

XIII. Limber Leg—Lie on your left side with your bottom leg out straight. Rest on your left elbow and upper arm. Draw your right leg in toward your chest and then extend it straight in front of you. Proceed to bring your knee in toward your chest again but while doing so rotate it so that your knee now points to the ceiling. Now raise your right leg straight above you (you might want to hold your right ankle to insure straightness) and return it to the flexed (knee bent) position before you rotate it down to begin a series of 20 of these combined kicks. When these kicks are completed, flex your bottom leg to help stabilize you while you tilt your pelvis forward a bit. Raise your straightened right leg up and slightly to the back of you as far as you can. While holding it there, bounce it 20 times and then flex your knee and attempt to touch your toes to your buttocks. Extend your leg again and repeat, touching your buttocks 20 times. Lie on your right side and repeat the entire sequence.

XIV. Arc of a Diver—Lie face down on the floor with your hands under your pelvis and your face forward. Your legs should be spread about 18 inches. Now lift both legs as far as you can off the floor, keeping them straight. Lift your chest off the floor. Touch your heels together eight times. Do not stop while you proceed to scissor-kick your legs, crossing first to the right over the left then spreading them and crossing the left over the right. Do this eight times. Repeat the sequence four times. Relax momentarily by resting flat on the floor, then continue with another set of the same.

Nosey Knee

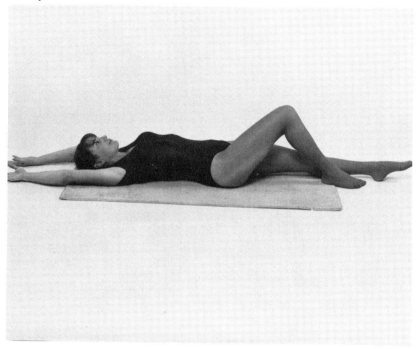

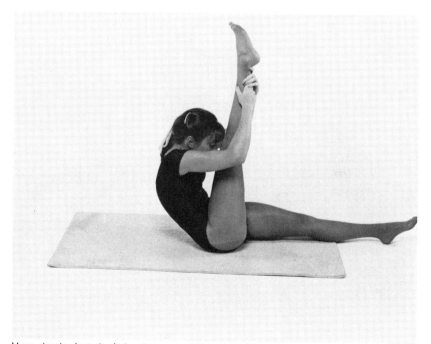

Very simple, but don't be discouraged if you can't touch your nose to your knee the first time; do it as well as you can. It'll come.

Back Bend

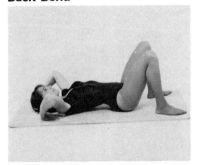
If your back is bad, skip this one.

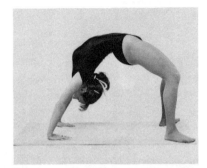
Raise yourself as high as possible.

Straight Leg

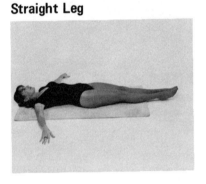

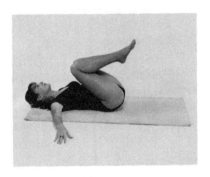

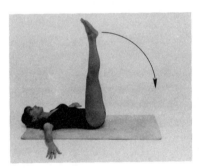

This is much easier than it looks. Bring your knees to your chest, and raise your legs toward the ceiling, lowering your straightened legs slowly to the floor, but not quite touching it. The picture below starts the next portion of the sequence, which is literally the same as the first, but done from a position holding yourself up on your forearms.

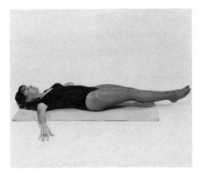

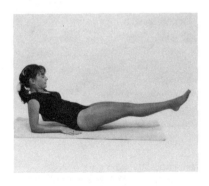

cont'd next page

Straight Leg (cont'd)

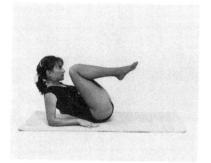

The sequence, as we've already stated, is the same as the first sequence was, the difference being that you're working the muscles differently because you are up on your forearms, thereby using your lower back more.

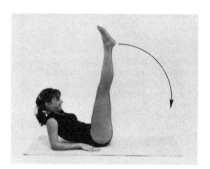
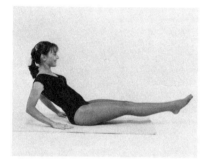

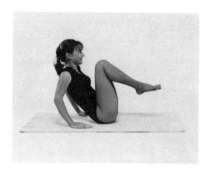

This is also the same sequence, but again, from a different angle created by raising your body up on your extended arms. Make all the movements smooth and controlled, and keep the legs together at all times.

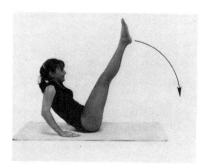
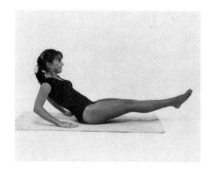

Limber Leg

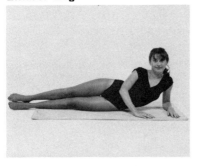
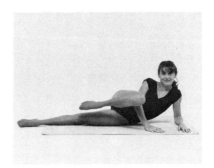

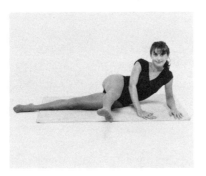

This is one of the easiest exercises in this entire sequence. Lie on your side, keeping your lower leg straight, and supporting yourself on your lower elbow, and obtaining additional balance from placing your free hand on the floor in front of you. Then, bring the upper leg forward, bending it at the knee; then straighten it; bring it back, rotate it, and turn it toward the ceiling; straighten the leg.

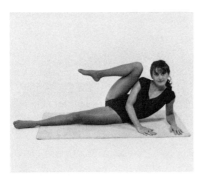
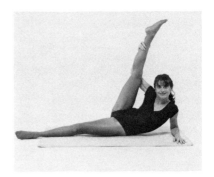

Arc of a Diver

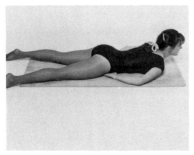
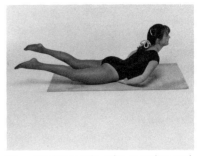

Lie face-down on the floor, with your hands under your pelvis, legs 18 inches apart.

Now simultaneously raise your legs and your chest as far as they will go.

cont'd next page

Arc of a Diver (cont'd)

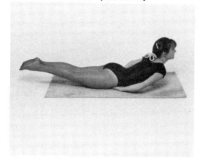

Now, bring your feet together in a clap; repeat eight times. Then begin a series of alternating scissor-kicks, repeating the kicks eight times. This should not be overdone if you have a weak lower back.

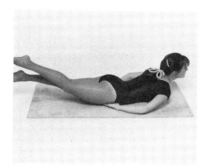
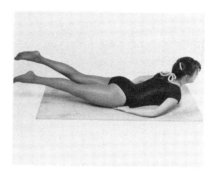

XV. The Essential Pushup Plus a Walk—Lie flat on the floor with your face down. Rest the palms of each hand flat on the floor beside their respective shoulder. Keep your legs and back straight and proceed to do 20 pushups, lifting your entire body off the floor while keeping it perfectly straight.

When you have completed the pushups, continue to hold yourself off the floor and continue to keep both your arms and legs straight while first you "walk" with your feet to your hands and back, and then "walk" with your hands to your feet and back. Keep legs straight at all times.

XVI. The Knee as Foot—Kneel erect, holding your tummy in and your arms out in front of you parallel to the floor. Continue holding your arms out straight while you drop to sit on the floor to the left side of your feet. Without the aid of your hands, resume your kneeling position and proceed to drop now to the right side of your feet, again holding arms out straight in front of you. Return again to the kneeling position and repeat this sequence 20 times.

When you have concluded this portion, sit back on your feet and grasp your ankles with your hands. Thrust yourself forward and attempt to achieve a standing position—on your kneecaps. You will need to draw your feet to your buttocks to do this properly. Test your sense of balance once you have gotten up by trying to walk on your knees. A word of caution: Do not attempt to do this on a hard surface—your knees will not appreciate it!

XVII. Standing Back Bend (a.k.a. The Fly)—Stand with your back against a wall. Now, walk out from the wall the length of two of your feet. Plant your bare feet on the floor, making sure you are not on a slippery surface, such as a rug. Now, very carefully and smoothly, reach your hands over your head and back to the wall. When you make contact, place your palms on the wall, and begin "walking" down the wall until your hands touch the floor. Pause a moment, and walk back up the wall.

This should not be an extremely difficult exercise/stretch if you are properly advanced. If, on the way down, you feel you are losing it, stop where you are, and roll to either side, until you face the wall. If you have a bad back, don't try this one at all.

The Essential Pushup Plus a Walk

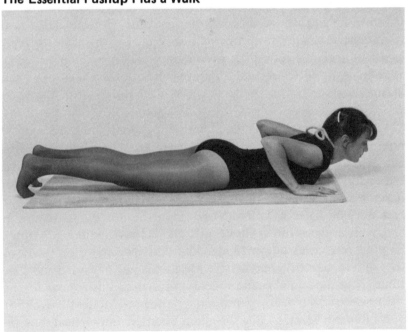

Lie flat on the floor, legs straight, toes to the floor, arms beside your chest.

cont'd next page

The Essential Pushup Plus a Walk (cont'd)

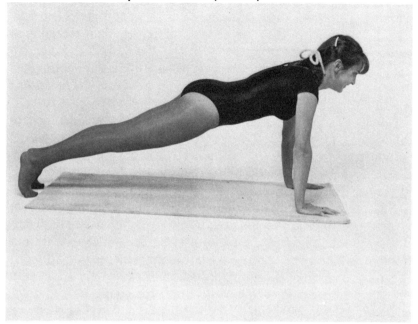

The back and legs should be kept straight; all "work" should be done by the arms.

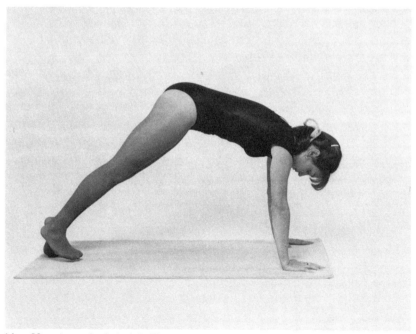

After 20 push-ups, begin jack-knifing yourself, as you begin to walk forward.

cont'd next page

The Essential Pushup Plus a Walk (cont'd)

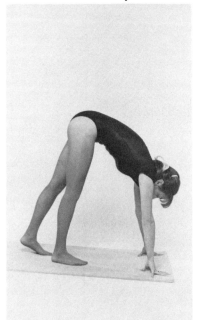

Continue walking, keeping hands on floor.

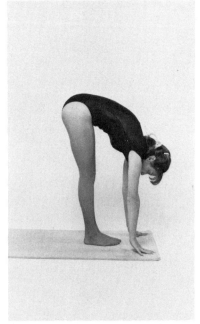

When your feet reach your hands, stop.

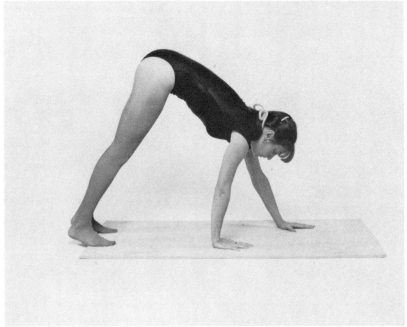

After walking back with your feet, begin to walk with your hands toward your feet.

cont'd next page

Floor Games 189

The Essential Pushup Plus a Walk (cont'd)

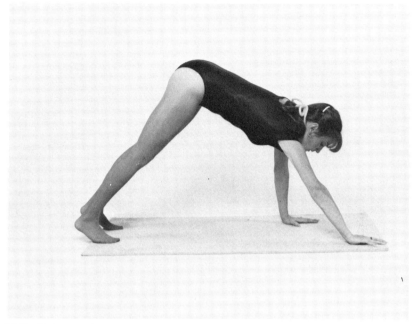

Walk all the way back to the jack-knife position. Repeat the walk at least once more.

The Knee As Foot

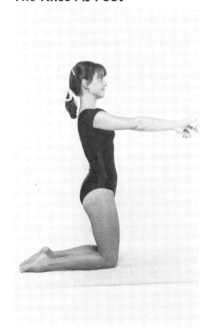

Begin by kneeling erect, with your arms out in front of you.

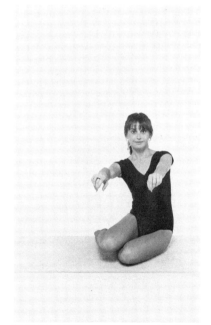

Continue holding your arms out in front of you and sit down on your left hip.

cont'd next page

The Knee As Foot (cont'd)

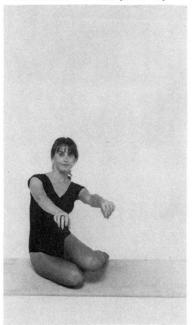

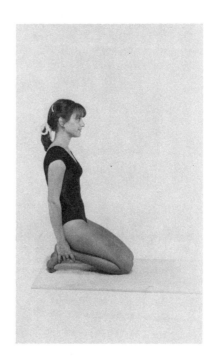

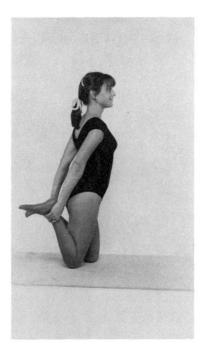

Without the aid of your hands or arms, keeping them out in front of you, resume your kneeling position and then drop to the right side of your tucked-in feet, resting on your hip. Return to the kneeling position. Repeat the exercise sequence 20 times. Then grasp your ankles with your hands and begin to walk back and forth on your knees. This takes some practice, but can be fun once you've mastered it.

Standing Back Bend

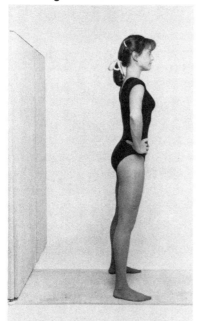

Stand with back to wall, about two feet away.

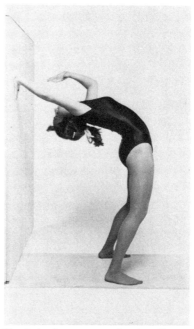

Reach back over your head until you touch the wall.

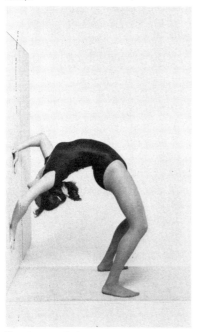

Slowly, carefully, walk yourself down the wall.

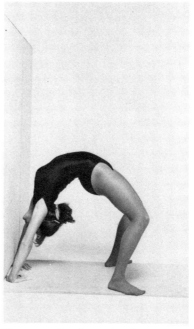

Plant your hands on the floor behind you. Walk back up.

Now take a breather and read the next chapter.

6

The Muscle Beach Party Gang Meet Slim-Person
by Richard Benyo

There comes a moment in the life of each boy when muscles are discovered. It arrives about the same time he discovers girls. He soon learns that there are at least some girls who are attracted to boys because of their muscles—or are at least gleefully impressed by them. Spurred by this influence, he begins to think seriously about growing some muscles of his own. There is a great moving force at work during that portion of the boy's life, because he is usually a freshman in high school, and being a freshman has often been called "the lowest form of life known to man." By growing a few muscles, he can usually soften the sharp edges of getting through his freshman year.

With the dual incentives of impressing the girls and defending himself against vicious sophomores, it is no wonder that some 15- or 16-year-old boys become muscle-obsessed, which is a variation of muscle-bound. Muscle-obsessed affects the brain.

Muscles are very impressive to a kid during his first year in high school. Everyone who is anyone seems to have bigger and stronger muscles than the 15-year-old kid, and he quickly learns that in many situations those with big muscles will get what they want, whether it's the prettiest girl in class, a position in the front of the line to the Saturday night movies, or a spot on the sidewalk previously occupied by someone with lesser muscles and not enough cheek to bluff out the bulky guy. Muscles make everything happen in the 15-year-old's world, because the 15-year-old's world is still largely physical and not mental. Muscle-power produces immediate results: brain-power takes a little longer to get the job done.

Two of my 15-year-old friends became very interested in muscles. In both cases, they had older brothers, who had also been interested in muscles. If you have an older brother who is into muscles, you also must become interested in muscles, for two reasons —self-defense and revenge. Older brothers have a habit of trying out their new muscles on their younger brothers. This must be a trait common to the animal world, because older, parental animals nip and scratch and roll their offspring around to teach them certain movements and defenses against enemies that they'll face in the outside world. I think that older brothers are supposed to do that, too. It's nature's way of passing on some of what they learned to their younger brethren so that he doesn't have to learn it wll the hard way. Of course, the younger brother never sees it that way, and he attempts to protect himself from the nips and the abuse, and in dark corners of his room, late at night, he stays awake an extra half-hour plotting revenge upon his older brother. The revenge seldom comes, because the older brother somehow always stays one step ahead of his younger brother. But the self-defense can be developed—by buying and building muscles.

You see, you don't just magically develop muscles. There was an entire ritual 20 years ago. First you read every word of the Charles Atlas ads on the back cover of comic books. The famed ads show a 98-pound weakling at the beach getting sand kicked in his face by a big bully. The weakling writes to Charles Atlas, the Tarzan-like guy at the bottom of the ad who never seemed to age and who promised to turn the 98-pound weakling into a strapping young man who could give the big bully a dose of his own sand the next time he came by to antagonize him in front of his girlfriend. All of the story took place in a few artist's panels, but in actuality, it took much more time than that to develop the necessary muscles. And even longer to learn how to use them. But before you could officially begin to develop muscles, you had to buy these: a Charles Atlas course, a set of York Barbells and some muscleman magazines—a commitment to having muscles and using them, for right, justice and the American way.

None of us had much money, so our first move was one of revenge. We stole some muscleman magazines that my friends' older brothers had secreted under their mattresses.

In possession of a half-dozen muscleman magazines, we'd zip down local mountain trails to our hideout and we'd pore over them, examining biceps and triceps, bulging muscles and huge veins. We'd Christmas shop through the ads for chromed, glistening weight sets and vitamin and mineral and protein supplements that came in uniformly bland-colored packages but that seemed to offer so much more than our tame and parental-approved One-a-Day vitamins. If wishing could have made it so, several kids squatting in those cool, shaded, wooded paths would have burst through their polo shirts just like the Incredible Hulk, and would have gone on a rampage, pulling trees out by the roots and avenging themselves on all the older kids who'd picked on them over the years. It would have been a bloodbath. Kids who are 15 years old have that much vengeance stored up in them.

Although all three of us had part-time jobs, none of us were earning enough—much less saving enough—to even think about buying a set of real weights. We had many kid-type operating expenses, including baseball and football cards, comic books, orange sodas or tall bottles of RC Cola, Saturday movies and such essentials. The weights cost way too much for us to even think about buying. Which didn't stop us from thinking about it anyway, of course. Kids' worlds are made up of improbable dreams.

We had come to the end of dreaming, though. *We had become kids of action.* If we couldn't come up with the money to buy weights or a gym set, we'd make our own. We split up the assignments. I'd get some rops and stuff and get to work on building a gym down in our hideout in the woods, while Mike and Groggs would start making a set of barbells out of buckets, a pole and cement.

Even for that, though, we would need money to buy the ropes, buckets, cement, and various other paraphernalia. And keep in mind that in those days, when you did something like that your parents suddenly became very suspicious and wanted to know all the details of your sudden enterprise and energy. Parental suspicion ran very, very high when the still, lazy days of summer vacation gave way to sudden activity.

We managed to mask much of what we were doing. The construction of the gym down in the woods moved along quite well. Any kid can buy rope and get away with it, and since it was down in the woods, there was no need to bring it home first. I strung rope between trees and hung enough from branches to hog-tie a herd of elephants. If we'd have bothered to paint them green, the woods would have looked like Tarzan's jungle empire.

Mike and Groggs were not having as much good fortune. They had purchased two buckets, a broomstick (they couldn't find a metal pole), and a bag of cement. They timed it to mix cement at Mike's house while his parents were gone, but mixing cement is, at best, a messy business, and leaves lots of evidence. That was complicated by their failure to go through the process twice (because there were two buckets in which they had to pour cement to anchor the broomstick, and you can't very well put one upside down if the cement isn't dry while anchoring the other end in the second bucket), and that each time, the process of cement hardening is not something that can be hurried.

Mike's father had one of those tubs in which you mix cement and Mike and Groggs were well into the mixing before they realized that they didn't know what proportion of sand to mix with the cement and water. They also didn't have enough sand, so they improvised by throwing dirt and stones into the mix, or whatever they could find. The mix lacked that smooth, milk-shake texture that properly mixed cement exhibits. It had become more like oatmeal with raisins.

Additionally, the process was taking longer than they had expected. And halfway through it, they finally *did* realize that they'd have to go through this twice, that filling one bucket and standing the broomstick up in it until the cement hardened was merely step one. They'd mixed enough cement for six or seven buckets, though. By the time I wandered up to see how they were doing, it was like a scene from *"The Little Rascals."*

Although they'd been relatively careful mixing the cement, some of it had spilled onto the grass, and it's difficult to pick up when it spills. I ran my sneaker through it, trying to blend it with the grass. They'd already filled the first bucket and the broomstick was standing up pretty straight, although their dirty hands had caked cement drops onto the pole. Some of the cement was hardening on the stick, and I could picture us having to wear gloves to lift the thing for fear or ripping our palms to shreds. I turned the water hose on the pole and sprayed off the clots of cement as best I could.

The mad masons were still stuck with about six buckets of cement they had no use for. Now cement, especially cement with dirt and stones in it, isn't something you get rid of by flushing it down the toilet.

"We could dig a hole and bury it," Mike suggested.

"Where can we dig and hide the location and where will we put the dirt we take out?" I asked.

"Maybe we could just carry the tub over there and dump it over the bank," Groggs said, pointing to the side of Mike's yard, where there was a dropoff to the next yard below. Mike's house was built on the side of a hill, as were all the other houses on his street.

"It'd run down into their yard," Mike said.

"Maybe we could carry it down into the woods and dump it," Groggs said, suddenly becoming enthusiastic about being the one to come up with the most suggestions, no matter how absurd they were.

"Na," Mike said. "That'd take us all day. These things weigh a ton."

"Well, we wanted weightlifting," I said.

That was the wrong thing to say, because Mike was becoming frantic. There were too many things he wanted to do with his summer and to end up being grounded for a month and spending it in the parlor watching *"I Love Lucy"* while leafing through the same comic books for days on end appeared to be a grim possibility.

But I suddenly had an inspiration!

"Why don't we just let things fall where they will, and tell the truth," I sputtered, gaining momentum. "We'll show your dad what we were doing, and we'll go beyond that. We'll even do more—"

They were both looking at me as though I'd lost my mind.

"Look," I said, "let's get some tools and dig around your mom's clothesline poles. They've been sagging a bit. We'll pour the remaining cement around the poles. That should anchor them better and then we'll clean out the tub before putting it back, and surprise your folks. We can tell them that we wanted to make weights and saw that the wash line posts needed fixing, so we decided to surprise them by doing both things. Won't that be great?"

They were still looking at me crooked, but the idea was starting to find support. "Yeah," Mike said, brightening, "the truth. We'll tell them the truth. We'll just mix it in with some fibs. Great! Let's go!"

In a moment we had more of Mike's father's tools out in the

yard and we were industriously digging around the clothesline posts. They *were* in pretty bad shape, and a concrete foundation seemed more like a good idea. Our modest proposal had now turned into an urban renewal project, and had taken on monumental proportions. Somehow, the extra cement exactly met the needs of the holes we'd dug. We rushed around, spraying water onto the tub before any of the cement turned to concrete. We cleaned the tools and put them back in the shed, and we sat down on a patch of lawn shaded by a tree, drinking Nehi orange sodas and congratulating each other.

When Mike's parents came home, they were dutifully impressed with our enterprise, and seemed genuinely happy with the work we'd done. They were gracious enough not to comment on how dirty the concrete was and that we'd failed to smooth it on top like professional masons do. They even asked to see how our weights turned out. Unfortunately, we'd forgotten all about them in our excitement to cover up our transgressions. We found our best-laid plans had come to rest. The cement, which had been watery to start with, had failed to support the broomstick, which had taken a 25-degree list. The cement had set by this point so it was too late to correct the problem.

Mike's father began laughing. "You're probably better off," he said. "Once you put the other bucket on, that broomstick would have snapped when you tried to pick up the thing."

He kept laughing, finding something increasingly funny.

"What, what, what?" Mike demanded. "What's so funny?"

"You boys went to all this trouble to make some weights," he said, "when your brother's old barbell set is somewhere in the back cellar under all that junk behind the washing machine. He's got a whole set of weights. Don't you remember? We drove all the way down to York to pick them up."

Mike shook his head, confused.

"There's a whole set of them in there and he hasn't used them in years. "I'm sure you could buy them from him for five bucks or for cleaning his room for a month."

Mike still seemed confused. "I still don't remember them," he said.

"You tried to carry some of them in the house and dropped them. They took a chip out of the tile in your mother's kitchen," Mike's father added.

Mike shook his head in the affirmative. It was all coming back.

We adjourned to the cellar and began digging through years of accumulated debris piled behind the washing machine. We were like the archeologists at the Egyptian tombs. We fould enough stuff to stock an ambitious garage sale (but of course, this was before the advent of garage sales), and every once in a while, one of us would exclaim over some piece of junk. Mike's mom stayed upstairs, apparently either too intelligent to go rooting through the mess or saving her energies to put everything back after we had found what we were looking for.

But sure enough, as we dug deeper we began unearthing bits and pieces of the old weight set, a five-pounder, two 10-pound plates, until it all began coming together. The *clang* and *clunk* of metal against metal must have sounded like someone had installed an iron foundry under the house. In no time we had a pile of weights that would keep any strongman happy. There was a barbell set and a dumbbell set with interchangeable weights. We were suitably ecstatic, and after lugging them up through the kitchen and out into the backyard, where the clothesline poles were suitably anchored into the ground, we took inventory. One 10-pound plate was missing ("I think he used it as an anchor for the boat," Mike's dad said, referring to a rowboat he kept out at a local lake.) and the Allen wrench was corroded onto the locking plate on the end of the barbell. We applied some Liquid Wrench to free it, and began hosing down the weights and drying them carefully, as though they were newborn kittens. Even Mike's father became enthusiastic. He began putting the dumbbells together. "Let's see how the dumbbell handles the dumbbells," he said. A relatively short man, Mike's dad was nonetheless built pretty well. It helps when you're the principal of the local grade school system like he was. He began going through some alternating arm curls, bringing up one dumbbell while the other was going down. He pressed his chin down onto his chest and knit his brow in concentration, as he monitored his breathing. His face reddened and his eyes bulged, but he kept pumping, pumping, pumping—his breath coming in hisses—while Mike's mother stood looking out the kitchen window, shaking her head sadly. His strength flagged as indicated by his arm muscles binding up badly. We then heard a change in his breathing, as though he were going to attempt, in one breath, to suck empty a giant-size chocolate malt. And on the next breath, he pushed both of the dumbbells directly over his head, arms perfectly straight, and then brought them slowly down toward his sides, his arms still perfectly straight. He held his breath and could see the effort took a mighty toll of him. With the weights at his knees, he dramatically opened his hands and let the weights fall with a thump to the grass.

"There," he said, red faced and in a wheezing breath. We applauded his effort. He bowed slightly and walked briskly into the house. Mike told us the next day that the poor guy spent the entire night totally immobile in his chair in front of the TV, moaning every few minutes, while he kept asking Mike's mom, "But why didn't you stop me when you saw me doing that?"

After he had made his unforgettable exit, we fell to messing with the weights. The Liquid Wrench had done its work; the Allen wrench was turning and we began adding weights to the barbell. We added so many weights that we couldn't budge it, and then began backing off the weights.

For the next several weeks we followed a crash program for building ourselves up. We spoke in excited voices about returning to school in September, and not being recognizable. We more closely examined the musclemen in the magazines, tracing veins up forearms, comparing them to what we imagined was our own burgeoning muscle bulk. We strutted and posed in front of each other, imitating the men in the magazine, imagining ourselves going to football practice in August with more muscles than we knew what to do with. After working up a sweat and exhausting ourselves under the weights, we'd spend a typically active summer day, and then rush back to get in one more weightlifting session before we went home for supper. Mike's brother, who had been happy to take the five dollars and invest it in gasoline for his car, came by periodically to give us a few pointers. He'd impress us with how much weight he could lift but then he was getting good workouts every day or so by pulling the engine from his car to further soup it up or overhaul it. The engine was out of the car more than it was in. He tried to back us off a little from the amount of weight we were using "It's more important to get the motions down first," he kept telling us. "Don't try to lift a million pounds one time; it's better to lift 100,000 pounds 10 times. You need that motion happening to your arms; that's where the buildup in the muscles comes from. If you just stand there grunting and groaning and don't move the weight, you might as well stand next to the house and try to lift that. You won't be good for nothin' but a sawhorse."

He firmly believed that you should work to bulk your muscles, because that was the fashion among people working with weights. But in his admonitions about lifting 100,000 pounds 10 times instead of a million pounds at once, he had voiced the basic tenet of strength-training without bulking. Less weights, more repetitions.

Our obsession, then, was to lift tall buildings, not to build strength to be able to run around them a hundred times without becoming exhausted. Times, in some ways, do change.

TODAY'S BULK

There was a period that we can blame—like we blame a lot of things—on the Vietnam War, when bodybuilding seemed to vanish. In the 1960s, it was the Charles Atlas influence. Then came the late-1960s and early 1970s and all of us were protesting this or that; bodybuilding was the farthest thing from our minds. The only time it seeped into our consciousness was during leap years when the Olympic Games would be televised, and we'd see the power lifters trying to give themselves hernias in front of the world's television screens for Mother Russia. Russians built like gorillas would bring impossibly huge weights up off the floor amidst terrific concentration and great grunts of effort, throw them up over their heads, hold them there while 50,000 flashbulbs popped and judges hurriedly scribbled notes and scores, and then they'd drop the things to the floor with a *thud* that had to be recorded at earthquake-watch centers around the world. The next day a newspaper story told about how the guy lived with his mother on a commune and how his hobbies were raising a rare strain of violets, crochet, listening to opera, and tearing rivets out of abandoned bridges with his bare hands.

Many of the guys I know who did go to Vietnam spent a good deal of their free time bodybuilding. Some of them came back with muscles they'd never had when I knew them. They contended that there was little else to do, and that you often tend to become obsessed with your body when you're not certain how long it will stay in one piece.

In the late-1970s and certainly by the early 1980s, a new mania for bodybuilding emerged. Some of it was due to *Pumping Iron* and some to *"The Incredible Hulk."* People—men and women both—became fascinated by the men who pumped iron as a steady diet. People mobbed famous bodybuilders (a.k.a., The Incredible Hulk and Conan the Barbarian), and felt their muscles, not always with permission, as though the guys were statues or livestock, or fresh fruit at the market.

The bodybuilding craze had its most dramatic leap when women became interested in giving it a try, as the decade of the 1980s dawned. The phenomenon of women bodybuilders got mass press coverage. Most of the major national magazines carried features on women's muscles, complete with full-color, full-page pictures of flexed female biceps. The national summer pastime of females going to the beach to ogle males strutting their muscles about had a dramatic addition. Now males ogled women bodybuilders as they posed in competition and in front of the cameras for feature magazines.

There is quite a physical difference between bodybuilding results for men and bodybuilding results for women. The difference is because of hormones that are unique to the sexes.

Whereas males who lift weights can bulk mightily, developing huge muscles with ragged edges, intertwined with veins and arteries that look like garden hoses, females who lift weights find that their muscles become more defined, but they do so with much more smooth, streamlined characteristics. There are very few visible ragged edges when a female flexes in a bodybuilding contest, although there are regimens that can be used to develop some ragged edges in women bodybuilders. She appears to be somewhat more *defined* but all the lines gently run into other lines. The male hormones that make overworked muscles begin to bulk are not present in her body, and the weightwork does not have the stark, almost alienating effect upon the body that males obtain.

Males who are into bulking through weightlifting are almost frightening to contemplate. Some people think the muscle-bound look is a thing of beauty. I'm afraid that I can't agree with them. I think that too much in flexibility and mobility is given up for the sake of maximum bulk. Aerobic advantages from bodybuilding (unless the person engages in an extensive program of aerobic weight training) are extremely limited. There is little advantage to the heart, lungs and the circulatory system, because there is little sustained activity: it is all bursts of exertion followed by extended periods of recovery, followed by periods of preparation for the next burst.

This is not to say that I'm against bodybuilding. If people want to spend all of that time—and it does take hours of work a day to maintain and build the body—and have a Charles Atlas body, more power to them.

It is becoming more apparent all the time, however, that endurance-type strength has more far-reaching advantages for the individual. If you like analogies, I suppose you could say that the difference between the bodybuilder and the endurance athlete is the difference, in auto racing, between the fire-breathing dragsters that make their run in six seconds or less, and the quick, nimble sports cars that compete in the 24 Hours of Daytona.

Personally, I'd rather go long than go fast and be finished quickly.

It is unfortunate that over the years, because of the bodybuilding image associated with weight work, the whole discipline has received an image that working with weights adds bulk. Nothing could be farther from the truth. A sensible weight program can build strength without adding bulk. In fact, a sensible weight program can actually cause you to lose inches—but not necessarily pounds.

WORKING FOR STRENGTH

The secret behind weight training is related to the theory of relativity.

What happens to your muscles when you lift weights will depend on how much weight you are working with relative to your body weight.

In other words, if you weigh 150 pounds and you bench press 120 pounds, you'll begin developing strength *and* bulk, and you'll be able to do the press a limited number of times.

However, if you weigh 150 pounds and you bench press 50 pounds, you'll begin developing strength *and* tone, and you'll be able to do the exercise several times in one session without a great deal of trouble.

The key is this:

Much Weight X Few Repetitions = Bulk

Limited Weight X Many Repetitions = No Bulk

For the person getting seriously into exercise who wants to concentrate on the mobile, endurance activities, a weight program using small weights and many repetitions is the answer.

Any bulk that you develop is merely extra weight that you must carry around during your chosen activity. If you are running for an hour on the treadmill and you have developed bulky muscles that add 20 pounds to your frame, you've lugged that extra baggage around for that hour.

The purpose of a good exercising program (whether indoors or outdoors) is to develop stamina, endurance, muscle tone, lose excess weight and build the heart, lungs and circulatory system. Taken to its ideal, what you are working toward is to move as effortlessly as possible, for as long as possible, as comfortably as possible, as often as necessary. And careful weight training can significantly contribute to that perfection.

Runners and cyclists are notorious for building stupendous endurance in the legs, heart and lungs. The strength in their legs is legendary. A 200-mile bike race? Why not? Running for 24 hours on a track? Can do.

Many of those same athletes, however, have relatively little upper body strength. And, to someone aiming for total fitness, and who wants to do well in his sport, strength and endurance must be built into all systems of the body—including the upper body.

Laboratory research shows that 10-12 percent of a runner's efficiency can be accounted for by proper arm strength and arm swing. If you're running a marathon, having upper body strength can significantly compensate for your not being able to maintain power in the upper thighs, which tire first in an extended run.

The importance of upper body strength is especially so for 400- and 800-meter runners. Watch them as they move around a turn; their arms are swinging and pumping. The arms provide both balance and strength, and the rhythmic arm swinging can measurably increase the stride of a runner in a short race or at the end of a long race when he is surging for the finish line.

Strength training, of course, is the backbone of almost every health club program. We've repeatedly talked about the sweating, intimidating giants working out on the Universal machine in the mirrored rooms. They are building strength and bulk.

It is easy enough to have a spindly runner reset the weights on the same machines and do a very vigorous workout that builds strength and does not add bulk. And he can do it in less time than the bulk-builders; he pumps iron while the bulkies are recovering between bursts.

YOU CAN GO HOME AGAIN

The answer, of course, is to abandon the Universal Gym at the health club and come home, either to your very own strength-training apparatus or to one that you've improvised.

You do not have to make a substantial monetary investment to have a functional strength-training center in the home. There are probably more unused weight sets around the country than there are big-wheel tricycles. Hit the Saturday garage sales one weekend and you'll probably be able to pick up a weight set dirt cheap.

A very simple, used weight set is more than sufficient for your purposes. It doesn't even have to be a complete set. If a few weights are missing, it's not the end of the world. You're not going to want to use a great deal of weight with each exercise anyway. If you are really creative and want to make a mess in your backyard, you could also do the trick with a steel pipe and two buckets and a bag of cement, but I don't really recommend that one.

You can, of course, avoid all the hassle and order an exercise station such as the one that is offered by The Wilson Design Group, marketed under the name SoloFlex. The unit is built specifically for the home, and has no bulky weights that make it a real project to assemble or move. The entire unit is based on resistance against graded bands. Much like large rubberbands, the bands (called 'rings') are placed on bars between the moving parts, and they make it progressively more difficult to move the apparatus as you ad bands or rings to it. The bands are coded with stripes that give you the weight equivalents. They are as follows:

$$1 \text{ stripe} = 12 \text{ lbs.}$$
$$2 \text{ stripes} = 25 \text{ lbs.}$$
$$3 \text{ stripes} = 50 \text{ lbs.}$$
$$4 \text{ stripes} = 100 \text{ lbs.}$$

Of course, you can use several of the bands and get various combinations. The SoloFlex is also built so that you can place free weights on it and use them as an integral part of the apparatus (up to 500 pounds), but its design is primarily for home use and for escaping the need for all those various-size weights sitting around and taking up a lot of room.

MAKING THINGS SIMPLE

Since there is so much mystery and ritual surrounding weight-type exercises, much of which combines to intimidate someone, we'll do away with all of the nonsense surrounding it and set down a few points. Then we'll get into a few basic exercises that you can do on a regular basis, at your own speed and convenience.

We'll make a few points first:

1) Never work with more weights or resistance than you can conveniently handle. Your weight work should offer resistance to your muscles, without strain or injury. This entire program, remember, is built on repetitions, and not on power lifting. The object is to strengthen, not to bulk. If you find that the weights or resistance you've set are difficult to lift or move, cut back. You should be able to comfortably move the weights. The benefit comes as you tire after lifting the weight seven or eight or nine times, not after getting hernias and not lifting it once.

2) As with any program of exercise, in the beginning certain "dormant" muscles will be used. Consequently, there will be some initial soreness, especially if you tend to push yourself. In order to avoid acute muscle soreness when you start the exercises, do not assume that they are extremely easy. They are *relatively* easy, and are in no way complicated, but they are still exercise. It will be much more comfortable for you if you ease into the exercises, making them a *part* of your other exercising, and not approaching them as if they are a challenge. They should not be a challenge. Soreness should not be a reason, if you begin the weight work sensibly, that you couldn't do a sequence seven days a week from the first day onward.

3) If you do develop muscle soreness, there are two ways to treat it. One is to come right back the next day and repeat the exercises, being careful to do them gently until the soreness works itself out, or you can skip the next day's workouts and hope that your muscles will have recovered by the second day. As long as you have not pulled and/or injured a muscle, working out with sore muscles will probably be more beneficial than bad. A light workout will loosen tight muscles, and it will get you through the "breaking in" period faster. If it is apparent when you try to repeat the exercises the next day that you have injured yourself, even if very slightly, immediately lay off the damaged muscle group and give it time to heal. Injuries don't heal by being worked back into shape; working an injury further aggravates it.

4) Try to work in your weight sequences either before or after whatever other exercising you're doing. Doing one workout session at a time rather than several workouts in a day has several

benefits. The most obvious is that the session keeps the muscles warm and loose for the next exercise, and the 24 hours that pass until the next workout will allow the muscles to heal and recover. Exercising two and three times a day puts your body under almost continuous strain, and allows no healing time.

5) If you are doing your exercises in the morning, do not jump right out of bed, sit down on the SoloFlex bench and begin doing bench presses. Give your body at least a half-hour of warmup and moving around before training. After sleeping, your muscles will be stiff and less flexible than later in the day. Also, don't do your exericses immediately before going to bed, because your muscles and body systems are slowing down in preparation for sleep. If you start doing exercises, you're stimulating your muscles and the rest of your body; you'll need another hour or two to calm yourself enough to sleep.

6) Don't engage in any vigorous exercise immediately after eating. This includes everything from running for an hour on the treadmill to making love. Your stomach signals the brain when it is filled, and that it has a lot of goodies down there to be processed. The brain accommodates by shunting a great deal of blood from other parts of the body (including the extremities, which are almost always intimately involved in exercise) to the stomach so that digestion can be accomplished. After a big meal, you should relax and allow the stomach to do its work. It isn't even a good idea to think too hard after eating (such as taking an exam), because some of the blood helping the stomach function is being diverted from the brain and you therefore are not at your sharpest upstairs. Give the stomach three to four hours to process the food. As the stomach tapers off its activities, the borrowed blood will be returned to where it was being used originally. If you exercise strenuously following a full meal, with all that blood preoccupied, the heart must work overtime to meet your demands.

7) When doing workouts on the treadmill, a good pair of running shoes is advisable, both because they will support and protect your feet, and should you decide to move your running outside, you'll be set with a good pair of shoes. Just about any shoe can be worn on the exercise cycle, as long as it is comfortable and flexes well. When doing weight work, especially with a system such as the SoloFlex, where you won't drop a weight on your foot, it is advisable to do the exercises barefooted. Allowing your toes to curl around the edge of the board for support is good exercise for them, as is planting your feet directly on the floor for

support when doing upper body exercises on the apparatus.

GETTING TO IT

We'll outline the 21 basic exercises suggested by the SoloFlex apparatus, and with each one that is applicable to free weights we'll include an explanation. There is no sense investing in a SoloFlex if you have a set of free weights lurking under a pile of stuff in the garage. Remember to start your program with a minimum of weight, concentrating instead on repetitions.

1. Dorsi Bar Pull Downs

SoloFlex: Space hands evenly on the bar. On each rep, pull the lever down as far as possible. Your head should tilt forward on each pull down. As in all weight work, exhale on the effort stroke, inhaling as you release the effort. The muscles in your upper back should be doing all the work.

Free weights: There is no corresponding exercise using free weights, because the exercise is in the same direction as gravity.

Dorsi Bar Pull Downs

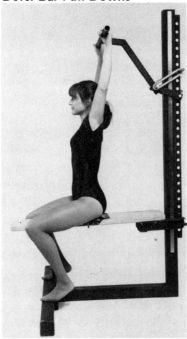

Keep your back straight and make every movement smooth and controlled.

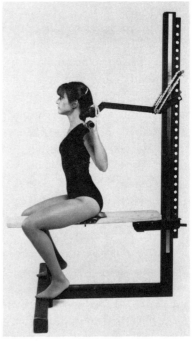

Pull the bar down toward your shoulders, using only the arms.

2. Press Off Back of Neck

SoloFlex: These take some getting used to. Begin slowly until you are comfortable with them and have built a firm foundation. Sit straight on the bench, and imagine a vertical line through your body. When you push up with your arms, keep them sliding up along that vertical line. Concentrate not on increasing resistance, but on your form. Again, exhale when you push up and inhale when you come back to your original position.

Free weights: Sit comfortably and straight on a padded bench. Rest the barbell on your shoulders behind your neck. Concentrate on making your upward movement smooth, straight and effortless. Push the weights toward the ceiling and pause at the top end before bringing them back down.

Press Off Back Of Neck

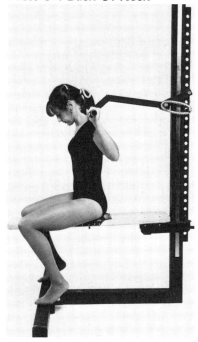

This is the reverse of the previous exercise; keep back straight.

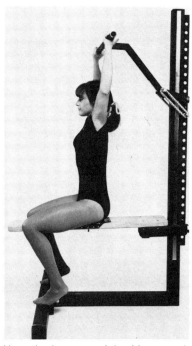

Use only the arms and shoulders to push the bar toward the ceiling.

3. Wide Grip Lat Rowing

SoloFlex: Sit directly under the handles, with your back and arms straight. Keeping your body straight, pull the handles down until they reach your chest, exhaling on the power stroke. Pause a moment, and return the handles to their original position, inhaling as they rise.

Free weights: There is no corresponding exercise using free weights, because the exercise is in the same direction as gravity.

Wide Grip Lat Rowing

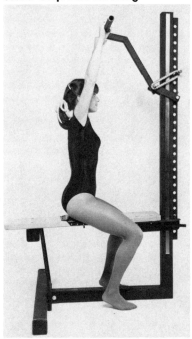
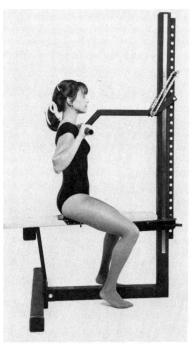

Make sure the bar is high enough to cause you to reach straight-armed.

Keeping the back straight, pull the bar down toward your chest.

4. Military Press

SoloFlex: Keep your back straight and sit directly under the handles. With an evenly spaced grip, push the handles toward the ceiling, holding them for a second at the top end, then return them to the original position. Exhale on the upward push, and inhale as you return the bar.

Free weights: This is one of the all-time standards in weightlifting. Sit straddling a comfortable bench. Keeping your back straight, hold the barbell against your chest. With your hands spaced evenly on the bar, concentrate on raising the bar toward the ceiling, keeping all movements smooth and coordinated. Do not use heavy weights. The movements and the reps are what is important. Exhale on the upward thrust, and inhale as the bar is returned to your chest.

Military Press

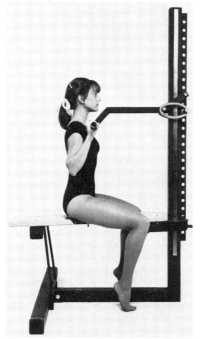

This is a reverse of the previous exercise; keep your back straight.

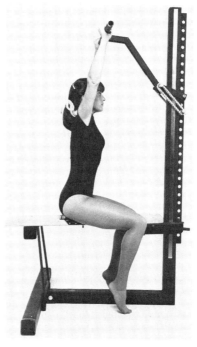

Push the bar toward the ceiling until your arms are straight.

5. Bicep Curl

SoloFlex: By doing a curl at this level and angle your normal effort is effectively doubled. Sit back a little from directly under where the bar will be when you pull it down. Grasp the bar from a palms-up angle, and smoothly pull it down toward your chest. Since the effort is nearly doubled, use a minimum of weights. Exhale as you pull it down, hold it at your chest for a second, and inhale as you return it to its original position. Never allow the bar, on one of the "pull down" exercises, to spring back to its original position; you should guide it back smoothly and have control.

Free weights: There is no corresponding exercise using free weights, because the exercise is in the same direction as gravity.

6. Bench Press

SoloFlex: Lying flat on your back on the bench, rest the bar on your chest and grasp it with hands spread at about shoulder width. Concentrating on smoothness, push the bar toward the ceiling, exhaling in the process. Hold it a moment and return it, inhaling on the return stroke.

Bicep Curl

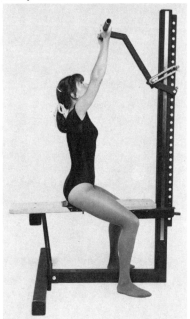 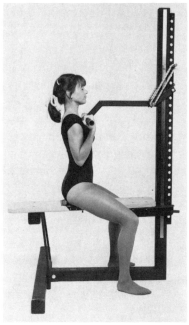

Grip the bar with an underhanded grip, and keep your back straight.

Pull the bar down toward your chest; feel the upper arms working on this one.

Bench Press

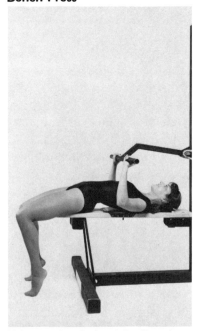 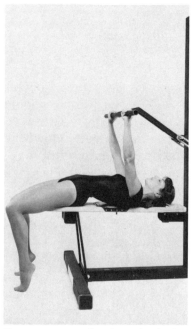

Make sure that the bench is adjusted to a point where it is comfortable.

Place your arms directly under the bar, and push it through the ceiling.

Free weights: This has always been one of the staples of weight-lifting. Lie on your back on a padded bench (a blanket over a wooden bench is fine), rest the bar on your chest using a grip that has your hands even with your shoulders, and push the bar toward the ceiling while exhaling. The secret is to always stay in control, keeping all movements smooth and coordinated. Pause for a second or two at the top end and return the bar to your original position. One of the major advantages of working on high reps and low weight, besides the fact that you can do the exercises in the comfort of your own home, is that you do not need a spotter, because you can easily control the weights. A spotter is someone who stands over a weightlifter, who is often lifting an inordinately big payload of weights, and sees that the weights don't fall on the lifter. If you are doing these exercises and even have an inkling that you need a spotter, you're working with way too much weight.

7. Bent-Over Rowing

SoloFlex: Use a very light weight. Be careful not to use your back in this lift. Back up against the upright, your butt against

Bent- Over Rowing

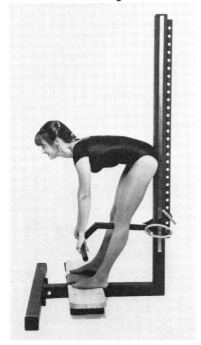

Place your buttocks against the upright; do not use your back.

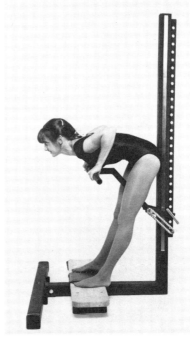

Do all the lifting with the arms, keeping the back immobile.

it. Keeping your head up, take a firm grip on the bar, your feet planted firmly on the crossbar. Smoothly pull the lever toward your crotch, exhaling as you do so. Pause, and return the lever to its original position, inhaling as you do so.

Free weights: You'll need additional apparatus on this one—a chair and a pillow. Place the pillow on the seat of the chair, face the front of the chair, and place your barbell (with minimum weights) in front of the chair on the floor. Bending at the waist and keeping your back straight, place your forehead on the pillow. Take a firm grip on the barbell, and pick it up vertically from the floor and bring it to your chest, exhaling as you do so. Pause a moment, and return the weight to the floor, inhaling as you do so.

8. Decline Press

SoloFlex: Standing on the crossbar and keeping your elbows out toward your sides, get above the bar and, using a smooth but forceful style, push the bar downward until your arms are straight. Keep your back in the same position throughout the exercise. All movement should be in the arms, using the chest muscles to help

Decline Press

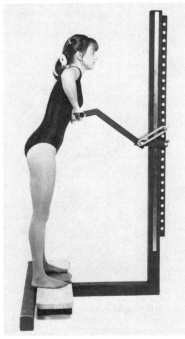

Make sure the bar is high enough so you must lift your elbows high.

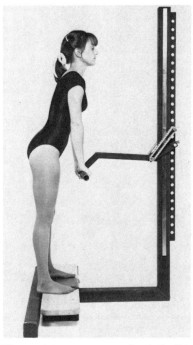

Then, using your arms only, push the handle toward the floor.

the arms exert the needed downforce. Hold the bar a second, and return it to the original position.

Free weights: There is no corresponding exercise using free weights, because the exercise is in the same direction as gravity.

9. Upright Rowing

SoloFlex: Form and not weight is very important in this exercise. Stand facing the bar, taking a grip approximately as wide as your shoulders. Keeping your back straight and unmoving, pull the bar up using only your arms. Hold for a moment, and return the bar.

Free weights: This one is extremely easy, but demands good form and coordination because the barbell should not touch you on the way up; rather, it should ride up a mere inch from your body. With an overhand grip on the barbell, allow it to rest at the length of your arms. Keeping your back straight, bring the barbell up to chest level using only the arms. Remember to exhale on the uplift, and inhale as you return it to its original position.

Upright Rowing

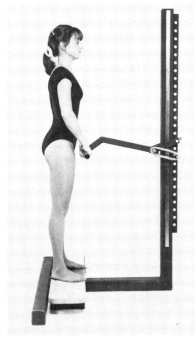

Set the bar at a height so that your arms are down level with your hips.

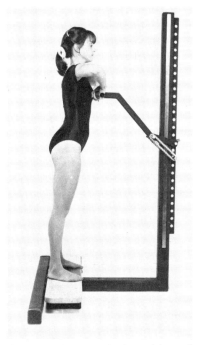

Then, keeping your back straight, pull the bar up with your arms.

10. Tricep Pushdowns

SoloFlex: Standing on the crossbar, keeping your back straight, take an overhand grip on the bar, elbows in tight. Carefully and smoothly press down on the bar, keeping your feet flat on the crossboard. Hold the bar down for a moment and then bring it back up.

Free weights: There is no corresponding exercise using free weights, because the exercise is in the same direction as gravity.

11. Tricep Extensions/Rear

SoloFlex: Stand on the crossboard, facing away from the apparatus. The position for starting this exercise is not an easy one to assume. It is easiest if you hold the bar down behind you while turning as you assume the starting position. Make sure all movements are smooth and controlled. Allow the bar to rise behind your back to your shoulderblades. Keep your feet flat. Press the bar down carefully. Be careful when dismounting; hold the bar down by directing the weight of your body through one arm as you turn to face the machine.

Free weights: There is no corresponding exercise using free weights, because the exercise is in the same direction as gravity.

Tricep Pushdowns

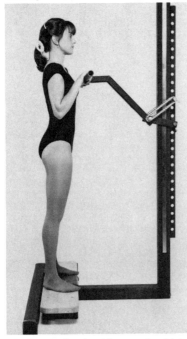

All the motion in this one should be centered in the arms.

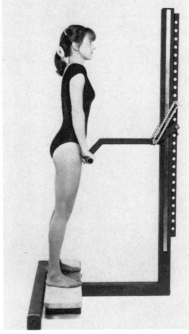

Keep your posture at its most perfect throughout the exercise.

Tricep Extensions/ Rear

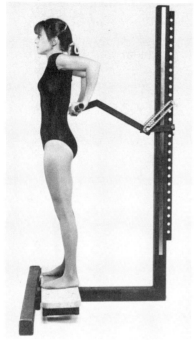
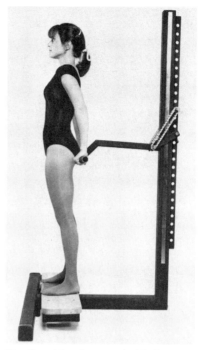

This one takes some practice in balance; do not set the bar too high.

Do all pushing downward with the arms, and do not bend the back.

12. Squats/Front

SoloFlex: Position the lever at waist height. Facing the upright bar, lower yourself under the handles, resting them on the deltoids. Keep the feet on the crossbar because when you push up you will be working against the machine and if you stand flat on the floor, you will lift the machine; by standing on the crossbar, you will be working against your own weight. Now, keeping your back straight and the handles positioned evenly, stand up and work against the resistance. The effort should be centralized in the legs.

Free weights: Standing straight, place the barbell across your chest, holding it in position by spacing your hands far apart on the bar. In a smooth motion, keeping your back straight and the bar fixed, bend at the knees and go into a squat. Pause a moment and slowly and smoothly stand up.

13. Squats

SoloFlex: Using the crossboard for support (and to hold the apparatus on the floor when you flex your mighty muscles), squat

Squats/Front

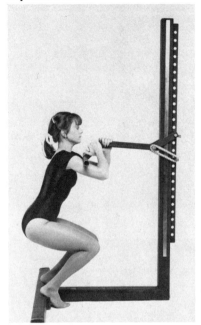

Squat with your heels on the bar and your toes on the floor, back straight.

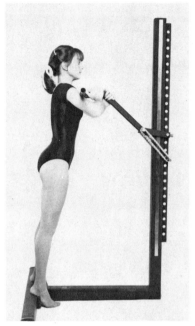

Keeping the back straight, merely stand up slowly but forcibly.

Squats

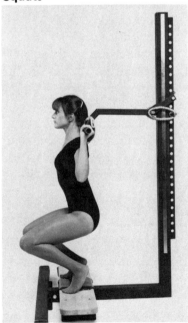

Use the cross-board on this one, and get up on your toes.

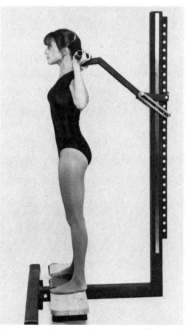

Then merely move into a standing position, being careful of posture.

down under the handles, resting them on your shoulders. (If this is uncomfortable, you can place a towel between the handles and your shoulders.) In a smooth, flowing motion, holding your back straight, stand up and work against the machine's resistance. Return to the squat position. Repeat.

Free weights: Standing straight, place the barbell across your shoulders behind your head and maintain your grip. In a smooth motion, keeping your back straight and the bar immobile, bend your knees and go into a squat. Pause a moment and then slowly and smoothly stand up.

14. Standing Calf Raises

SoloFlex: Stand on the edge of the crossboard, your back to the apparatus, with 60 percent of your feet (from the balls to the heel) over the edge. Push the handles up and place them on your shoulders behind your head. All movement centers in the feet and ankles. Once you are comfortable and balanced, raise yourself on your toes. Drop back to your original position with the heels over the edge of the board. Repeat, keeping the handles stationary.

Standing Calf Raises

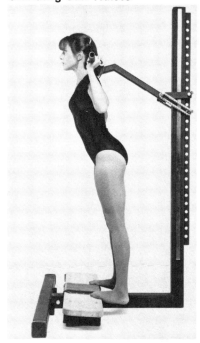 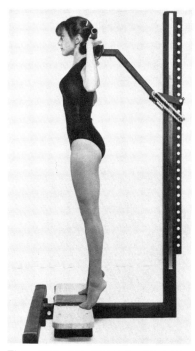

Stand with the toes on the board and the heels off.

Then push yourself up by using your toes; feel the calves work.

Free weights: This one is a little more difficult with free weights, because there is no stationary point of support, which is the inherent difficulty with using free weights. On either a step (the bottom one, certainly, so you can merely step off it if you begin losing your balance) or a board, stand on the edge, your toes on the step/board and your heels over the edge. Balance the barbell on your shoulders, behind your head, supporting it with your hands. Keeping every other part of your body straight and still, raise yourself on your toes, hold a moment, and lower yourself.

15. Donkey Press

SoloFlex: This exercise works primarily on the calves, one of most difficult set of muscles in the body to build because of its density. Increases in size and strength require increased stretching of the calves. With the bench attached, lay down on it, your head away from the upright. Push the handles up with your legs, keeping them straight. Make sure that the handles are being pushed by the balls of your feet (about 40 percent back from the tips of the toes). Now, with your knees straight, push the handle up and down using only your feet, as though the balls of your feet were the palms of your hands. All movement should be in your

Donkey Press

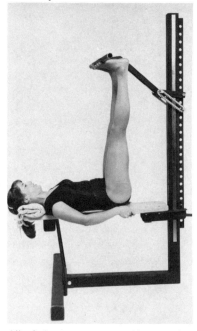

All of the movement on this one, also, comes from the toes.

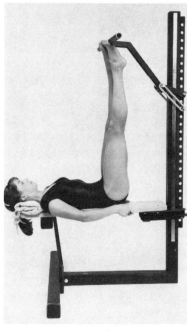

As your toes push the bar up, the benefit comes to the calves.

The Muscle Beach Party Gang Meet Slim-Person

ankles. This exercise will feel somewhat uncomfortable at first, and may even be painful. If it is, it's working.

Free weights: This exercise is almost impossible with free weights unless you are an experienced juggler and balancer. It's possible to do it haphazardly if you use a spotter, but isn't recommended because the weights could very easily roll off your feet and cause an injury. If you want to invest in a set of ankle weights, this exercise could be done by attaching the ankle weights around the front of your feet.

16. Leg Press

SoloFlex: Using the same position as you did in the Donkey Press, flex and straighten your legs against the resistance of the handles. Repeat, keeping your back comfortable and straight on the bench, supporting yourself with your hands. Attempt to extend your legs until they are perfectly straight.

Free weights: It is unsafe to attempt this exercise with free weights. If you have a friend, however, he can stand near your rump while you lay on the floor, and can lean his stomach into your feet, offering minimum resistance as you push him up and down. For your purposes, however, a friend's weight might be excessive.

Leg Press

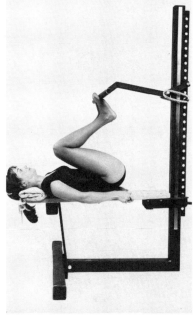

Place a towel or pillow under your head and grip the board.

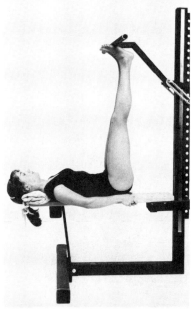

Using only the legs, push the bar toward the ceiling.

17. Dead Lift

SoloFlex: Stand on the crossboard, facing away from the apparatus and straddling the lever. This should not be done if you have a weak lower back or are prone to back pains, because all the lifting is done with the lower back. Bend down and grasp the handles with an overhand grip and in a smooth, careful motion, straighten up, bringing the lever up into the crotch. Concentrate on smoothness.

Free weights: Stand in front of the barbell and bend down, keeping the legs as straight as possible. Grasp the barbell at shoulder width. Using your lower back, straighten up, bringing the weights with you, exhaling as you do so. Return to your original position in one smooth motion.

18. Incline Press

SoloFlex: By tilting the bench up at the upright, you can get a completely different angle, which will help build the pectorals. With your feet planted on the floor, and with a wide grip on the handles, push the handles toward the ceiling, exhaling as you do so. Repeat.

Free weights: You can place a lift under the end of the bench to get the elevation needed. Support yourself by planting your feet firmly on the floor, and do basic bench presses.

Dead Lift

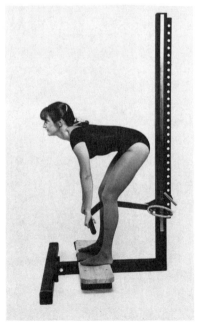

Make sure that the legs are bent, because that's where the strength is.

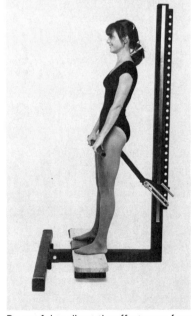

Be careful to direct the effort away from the small of the back.

Incline Press

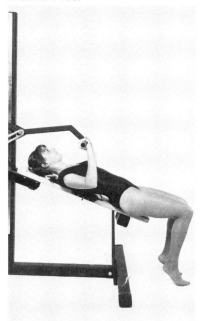

Support yourself on your toes for best effects from this one.

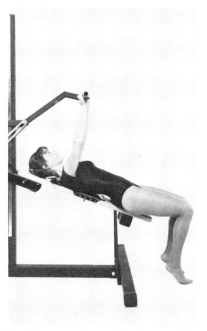

Use the arms only, pushing them straight up toward the ceiling.

19. Body Curls

SoloFlex: Slant the board at a shallow angle, placing your head near the upright, holding onto the upright for support. Keeping your legs straight, curl your legs toward the top of the upright, bending at the waist.

Free weights: You do not need weights to do this exercise. Put one end of your bench against the wall, adding a bit of lift under that end. With your head toward the wall, lay on the bench and grasp the edge of it near your head for needed support and then, with legs straight, raise them toward the wall, bending at the waist.

20. Incline Sit-Ups

SoloFlex: Tilt the bench at the edge away from the upright and using the anchor for the rings, put your toes under the anchor for support. Bend your knees 90 degrees, and put your hands behind your head, bringing your elbows up to touch your knees on each sit-up. Do not do them too fast. Control is important.

Free weights: This is difficult to do on a bench that sits there all by itself, because there is no place to anchor your toes for leverage. If you have a board, place it on the floor and raise one end. Lay down and rest your head at the lower end, placing your feet over the high end, bending the knees at 90 degrees. With hands behind head, proceed to do sit-ups.

21. Leg Bends

SoloFlex: With the bench slanted down at the end away from the apparatus, grasp the upright while laying on your back. Keeping your legs together, bring them up to your chest slowly and carefully, and just as slowly and carefully, return your legs to a straight position. Repeat.

Free weights: Place a small lift under the head of a bench, where your head rests, lay on the bench on your back, grasping with your hands the edge of the bench under your head. Straighten our your legs as though you're doing a dive into a pool. Bring your knees up to your chest, bending your knees as you do so that you go into a curl, keeping your legs together . . . . Hold for a count of two and return, keeping all movements slow and controlled.

Body Curls

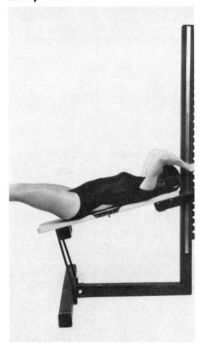
Grasp the upright to anchor yourself, and bring your legs up.

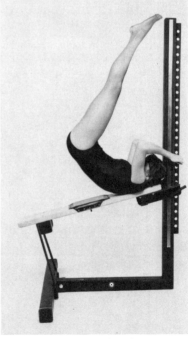
Keeping the legs straight and attempt to touch toes to upright.

Incline Sit-Ups

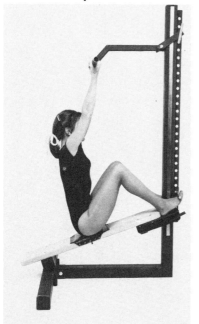

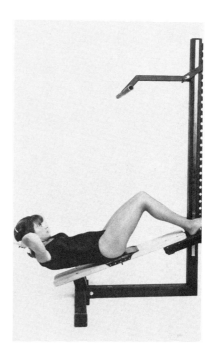

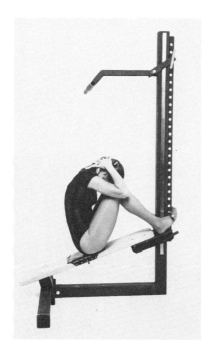

Use the bar as a support for getting yourself into the proper position for these exercises (upper left). Settle your buttocks onto the padded seat, curling your toes under the anchor on the upright. With your hands behind your head, and your knees bent, drop back into a horizontal position (upper right), from there touching your forehead to your knees.

Leg Bends

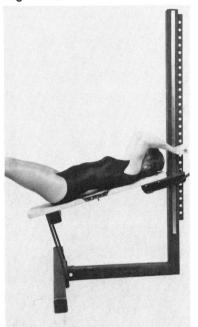

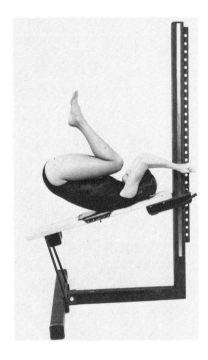

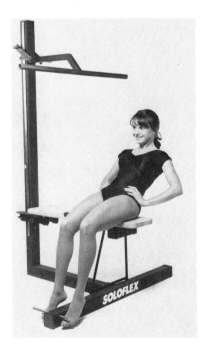

Settle yourself flat on the inclined board, grasping the anchor (upper left), then bring your knees up toward your chin (upper right), repeating the exercise. It's great for the abdomen. Another great one for the abdomen is to side side-saddle on the board, and use the anchor on the leg of the apparatus (left), essentially doing sit-ups without using your hands.

THE PACE PLACE

As in all the exercises we've discussed, the tendency—as with everything else today—is to want it all to happen *now*! When exercising, forget that idea. Exercising should not be a burden, a trail or a race. It should be well-paced, very patient and relaxing.

Do not turn your SoloFlex or your garage-sale free weights into machinery from the imagination of the Marquis de Sade. Stay at a specific level until you feel you have done all you want to do there. When dealing with the SoloFlex or weights, you have two different ways to push to the next level, and the two methods should never be used at the same time: 1) Add some more weight or resistance. 2) Increase the repetitions ("reps").

It is advisable to keep a journal or a wall chart of your workouts so that you can follow your progress. After a few months, you'll see a pattern of your workouts increasing in intensity. That progress should set your mind at ease, and then you won't feel so inclined to rush.

When you think you have stayed on a development plateau long enough, there are some rules to keep in mind before increasing your workload.

Your first consideration should be to consider adding weights. By judiciously adding weight, you can keep the same workout sequence, thereby not spending more time training. You can also save the program you've grown comfortable with. Remember, though, that you want to avoid bulking, so you must set weight limits. You should be able to comfortably do a minimum of a dozen reps and two sets of each exercise before considering increasing the weights. If you are doing one set of the exercises at 15 reps, but are having trouble getting through the second set, don't add either reps or weight. Stay at that level until it becomes comfortable to finish the second set. It just takes time.

If you are able to do a dozen reps of each exercise twice, and fully recover the next day, you can think about adding weights or resistance. Be conservative. Adding five pounds would be quite enough. In fact, the rule of thumb is not to add more than five pounds at a time. On the SoloFlex, that becomes complicated because of the way the resistance rings are graduated. Make the smallest possible increase on the SoloFlex and stay at that level for a few weeks. On the exercises where you are working against your body, and there are no weights involved (such as the Leg Bends), merely increase the reps.

If your program consists of all 21 exercises we've discussed, and you do two sets of 12 each, you are doing 504 reps, which is a formidable exercise program five days a week. That's 2520 reps a week. If you increase your reps by only "1" you will be effectively adding 42 reps per day, or 210 per week, raising your total for the week to 2730. Increasing your reps by "5" makes it 210 per day, 1050 per week, or a total of 3570 for the week. A jump from 2520 to 3570 is just too much.

So make your increases by "1" rep. In fact, if you have a progress chart on the wall of your training room, you might want to take some paper, write a big "1" on it, and hang it above your progress chart to remind yourself.

Go cautiously. Just so you keep going. Because as long as you keep moving, all the destructive things life throws in your path will be overcome. Everything, that is, except such broad-reaching statements.

It is tempting to end this book with some weighty or profound statement that will very neatly and cleanly bring together everything we've discussed. But that isn't what exercising and the active lifestyle is really about. This is what it is all about:

Keep moving so that when life tries to pass you by, you're already two steps ahead of it.

Or how about this one:

The unperspired life is not worth living.

Or how about . . .

About the Authors

Richard Benyo is execituve editor of *Runner's World* Magazine and editorial director of *Skier's World* and *Fit Magazine.* He authored several other books, among them *Return to Running* and *Superspeedway.* A veteran of many marathons and ultramarathons, he does flexibility and strengthening exercises following his daily training runs. Skinny in high school, Benyo swelled to two hundred seven pounds before he turned thirty, but came down to one hundred fifty-five pounds following a resumption of a resular exercise program.

Rhonda Provost is a nurse anesthetist from Boston. Her profession gives her a healthy background in medicine and science. She has been living the type of life she advocates for as long as she can remember. She currently resides in Palo Alto, California, where she is a member of a local health spa, runs, skis, and is an avid cyclist.

Benyo and Provost co-authored the *Runner's World Indoor Exercise Book* as their previous effort. Besides their interest in exercise, they collect and enjoy old rock 'n' roll records, enjoy hot-air ballooning, camping, and sampling the many wines for which California is famous.

Recommended Reading

The following books, also available from Anderson World, can augment your exercise and fitness program. They are available from major bookstores or can be ordered directly from the publisher (1400 Stierlin Road, Mountain View, CA 94043).

THE RUNNER'S WORLD INDOOR EXERCISE BOOK by Richard Benyo and Rhonda Provost. A beginner's guide to exercising in the comfort of your own home, where the mad dogs of August will not nip at your heels, where the automobile traffic will not attempt to give you that run-down feeling, and where the pollution will not make breathing an anaerobic exercise. The concentration is on building flexibility, endurance and strength, without bulking muscles. The logical introduction book on indoor exercise that prepares a person for the "advanced" book you are now holding in your hands. Spiral bound. $11.95.

RETURN TO RUNNING by Richard Benyo. As children, everyone ran as perfect moving animals, with no restrictions or restraints. Somewhere along the road to maturity, we loose that natural love of running. It can, however, be recaptured. The co-author of *The Runner's World Indoor Exercise Book* and the editor of *The Complete Woman Runner* tells the humorous story of how he went from 207 pounds to 162, moving from a desperate struggle to cover a quarter-mile to running the famed Boston Marathon. Fun reading for those who feel that running is probably too much for them, and for those who want to recapture that joy of movement that children seem to keep for themselves. Quality paperback. $3.95.

THE RUNNER'S WORLD YOGA BOOK by Jean Couch with Neil Weaver. An easy-to-follow guide to using the principles of yoga for stretching, strengthening, and toning the body, and a good book to graduate to after you've outgrown some of the exercise routines in *The Runner's World Indoor Exercise book.* Spiral bound.$11.95.

TOTAL WOMAN'S FITNESS GUIDE by Gail Shierman, Ph.D., and Christine Haycock, M.D. A good guide to choosing a fitness program that fits your needs, you goals, and your lifestyle, with special attention to what happens to a woman's body during physical activity. Quality paperback. $4.95.

TOTAL FITNESS BEGINS WITH THE RUNNER'S WORLD INSTRUCTIONAL SERIES.
Try It for 10 Days ... FREE

BEGIN YOUR TOTAL FITNESS PROGRAM TODAY
This one-of-a-kind instructional series is an innovative assembling of all you need to learn and enjoy on the way to total physical conditioning.
In your own home, you can master the ancient art of yoga ... eat better, feel stronger with a natural food diet ... massage stress and tightness from your weary muscles ... learn the fundamentals of weight lifting ... incorporate positive stretching into your daily workout ... and actualize total fitness with this complete instructional how-to series.
Every volume in the *Runner's World* Instructional Series is spiral-bound for easy application — designed to lie flat while you progress through our instructional programs. Each book is written by leading professionals and edited by the staff of *Runner's World*. You are assured of a format that is understandable and readable.

A 10-DAY FREE EXAMINATION OF EVERY VOLUME
Every volume in the *Runner's World* Instructional Series can expand your fitness horizons for a 10-day FREE examination. Here's how it works: If you decide to keep your introductory volume, we'll send you future volumes in the series approximately every other month — one volume at a time, always for a 10-day examination. You keep only the volumes you choose — there's no minimum number to buy — and you may cancel your subscription at any time simply by notifying us.
Beginning with the *Runner's World Yoga Book*, the series moves on to the *Indoor Exercise Book, Natural Foods Cookbook,* and more. Send for your introductory volume today.

EACH BOOK IN THE SERIES:
- Big 6½" x 9¼" format
- Spiral-bound for easy use
- Approximately 200 pages
- More than 150 photos and/or illustrations, all with easy, instructional, step- by-step formats
- Can be used with or without a partner
- Is specially priced at $9.95 ... a savings from publisher's retail price of $11.95
- Written by leading authorities and edited by the staff of *Runner's World*.

START YOUR QUEST FOR TOTAL FITNESS
FREE FOR 10 DAYS

☐ YES, I would like to take advantage of a charter subscription to the *Runner's World* Instructional Book Series.
Please send my introductory volume for a 10-day free examination. If I decide to keep my introductory volume, I will pay $9.95 plus shipping and handling. I will then receive future volumes approximately every other month. Each volume is $9.95 plus shipping and handling and comes on the same 10-day free examination basis. There is no minimum number of books that I must buy, and I may cancel my subscription at any time simply by notifying you. If I do not choose to keep my initial selection I will return it within 10 days. My subscription for future volumes will be cancelled, and I will be under no further obligation.

Name_____

Address_____

City_____

State/Zip _____

Mail to:
Runner's World Instructional Book Series
1400 Stierlin Road
Mountain View, CA 94043

NO POSTAGE
NECESSARY
IF MAILED
IN THE
UNITED STATES

BUSINESS REPLY CARD
FIRST CLASS   PERMIT NO. 364   MTN. VIEW, CA

POSTAGE WILL BE PAID BY ADDRESSEE

Runner's World Instructional Book Series

1400 Stierlin Road
Mountain View, CA 94043